Da Yan
Wild Goose Qigong

The 1st
64 Movements

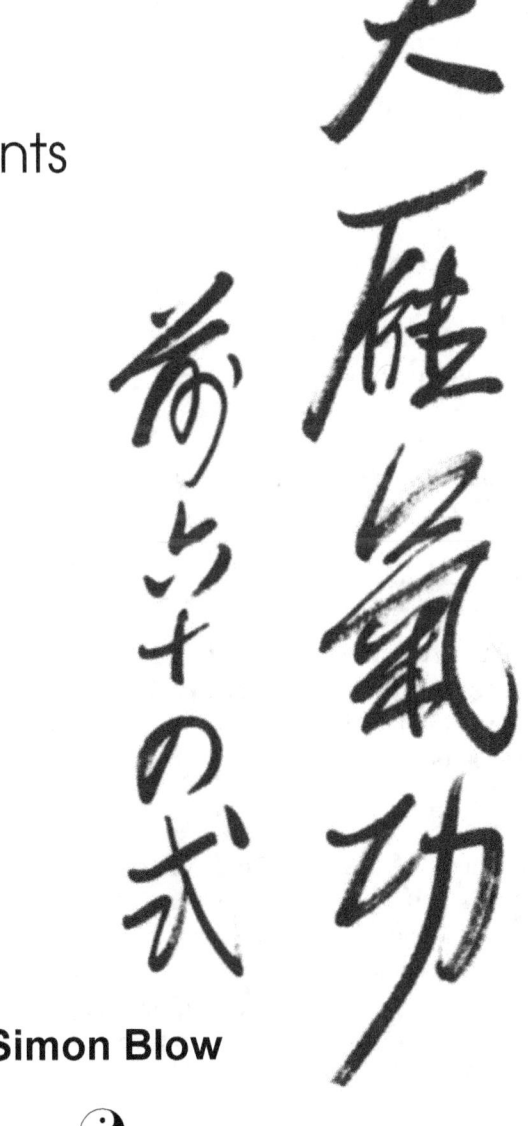

Simon Blow

First published 2014
Copyright © 2014 Simon Blow

National Library of Australia
Cataloguing-in-Publication data:

Da Yan Wild Goose Qigong – The 1st 64 Movements

ISBN: 978-0-9873417-6-1

Published by:
Genuine Wisdom Centre
PO Box 446
Summer Hill NSW 2130
Australia
(www.genuinewisdomcentre.com)

Editing:
www.essencewriting.com.au
www.mediawords.com.au

Cover design and layout:
Determind Design (www.determind.com.au)

Diagrams:
John Bennetts (www.johnbennettsmusic.com)

Disclaimer
The intention of this book is to present information and practices that have been used throughout China for many years. The information offered is according to the author's best knowledge and is to be used by the reader at his or her own discretion and liability. Readers should obtain professional advice where appropriate regarding their health and health practices. The author disclaims all responsibility and liability to any person, arising directly or indirectly from taking or not taking action based upon the information in this publication.

This book is dedicated to

To my parents Gordon and Joan Blow, for bringing me into this world, giving me love and support and allowing me to find my own path.

Contents

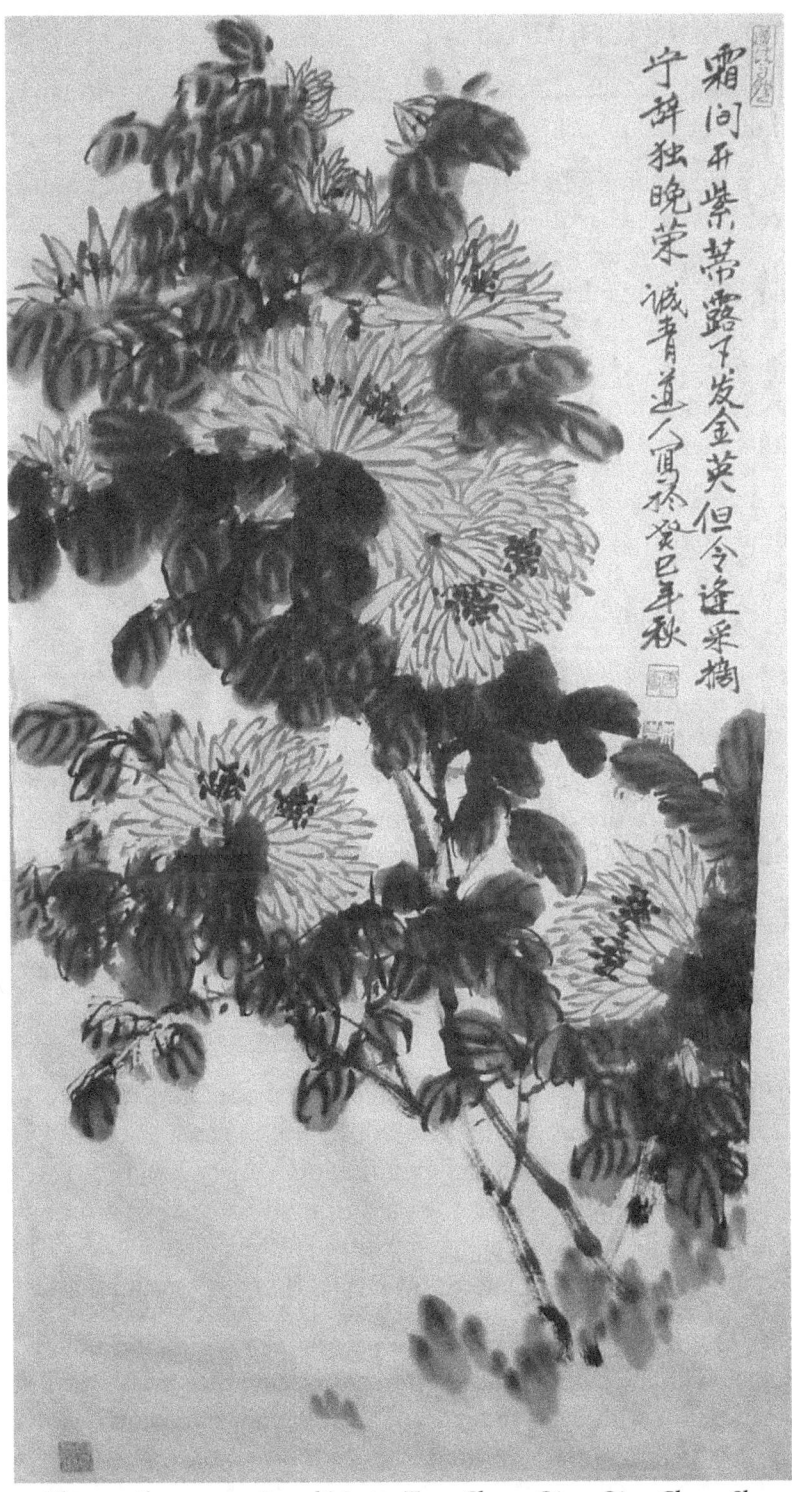

Chrysanthemums, Grand Master Tang Cheng Qing, Qing Cheng Shan
Green City Mountain, Sichuan Province, China. September 2013

Acknowledgements

There are many people I would like to thank for helping me to compile and develop this book.

Since I started teaching full-time in 1992, I have been teaching many classes each week for the general public and within therapeutic communities. I have had the great opportunity to meet many people on their own healing journey and I have been inspired by their stories. I get many ideas and positive feedback from all the people I meet and from those who have generously shared their own experiences in this book. I'm not sure if we have original ideas or if, when the heart opens and the Qi flows, we are simply all one. Again, thank you.

I would like to thank all who have attended my classes, workshops and residential retreats over the years. Also to those who have travelled with me to China. Without all your help and support I would not have been able to continue on this path.

My great appreciation to Grand Master Chen Chuan Gang and Madam Chen for sharing their wisdom and insight with me and for accepting me into the Da Yan Wild Goose family. I feel very honoured that they have given me the opportunity to write these books and document their family legacy so all can benefit. As we have discussed many times; it's all meant to be, it's destiny. A special thank you to Zhang Jing, my Daoist brother and business partner. You have educated me and enriched my life with your friendship and guidance, allowing me to gain a deeper understanding of Chinese culture. Your expert translations and assistance in introducing me to many esteemed masters has allowed me to grow and understand and share the complexities of this ancient healing art.

I would like to thank Lynn Guilhaus and Elizabeth Bond for proofreading and editing and for bringing this project to life. Thank you John Bennetts for the original photos and drawing adaptations; every diagram is a work of art. Master Zhang Cheng Cheng for the original Chinese writing and Grand Master Tang Cheng Qing for the beautiful paintings. Thank you to Mamun Khan and all his team from Determind Design for the layout and design.

We refer to Qigong as an art form. It is a process of refining our internal energy to harmonise with the external energy or environment. It's our own observation of our relationship with everything around us. We are influenced by everything around us; we are one with everything.

Foreword

'Simon Blow is an academic ambassador working for the cultural exchanges between China and Western countries. Over the past twenty years he has been to China many times, visiting the sacred mountains and holy areas in China while studying the ancient Chinese methods for health and longevity. He has made a life-long commitment to introducing and spreading these traditional Chinese health and wellbeing skills overseas.

'Simon first learned about the Wild Goose Qigong when he visited Wuhan in 2007. We met through a friend and since then he keeps coming to Wuhan every year, learning the Wild Goose Qigong from me. He was working so hard on every single movement. He thought the Wild Goose Qigong was among the best Qigong trainings for health. He really loves Wild Goose Qigong.

'As a student when learning, Simon respects his teachers and admires all the knowledge he is taught. He has made a great effort in learning, trying to make everything perfect. He never stops asking questions until all becomes completely clear. I am moved by his learning spirit. Simon has learned both the 1st and 2nd 64 movement set, the basic skills of the Wild Goose system. He has practised these skills over 3000 times and obtained an in-depth understanding of the secrets within the training through his dedication towards it.

'As a teacher when instructing, Simon is caring for every student. He is trying to make the complicated theory simple and easy for students to understand. He is leading the practice personally and repeating the difficult parts of movements again and again, to make sure that everyone can learn it properly. All students love his way of teaching.

'Simon brings his groups of students to China every year for refinement trainings with me. When he is leading the practice, he often asks me to stand aside to watch the students to see which movements they are not doing correctly. I can find their wrong postures easily in this way. In fact I seldom use this teaching method for my own students. I must admit that Simon is a brilliant Wild Goose Qigong Master. He is my best 29th generation lineage student overseas.

'To better spread and teach the Wild Goose Qigong (with the teaching principles of being genuine, accurate and honest), Simon is writing a book in English on Wild Goose Qigong with his own experiences and feelings as a reference. He has come to me several times to discuss, refine and finalise all the details on each chapter of the draft. This is the teaching textbook on Wild Goose Qigong in accordance with the original principles of the ancient masters. There are accurate instructions for all the movements, genuine meaning and interpretation of understanding, without any change or someone else's words added to it. This is the best version in English on Wild Goose Qigong I have ever seen. I hope all practitioners read it carefully.

'My congratulations on this book written by Simon. I wish Simon's teaching career of Wild Goose Qigong development becomes more successful.

'I wish the Wild Goose Qigong, this miracle training skill, flourishes with more students learning in all different parts of the world.

'We can work together for the Wild Goose Qigong cause, for the health benefits of all human beings on earth!'

Chen Chuan Gang, 28th Generation Lineage holder of Wild Goose Qigong.

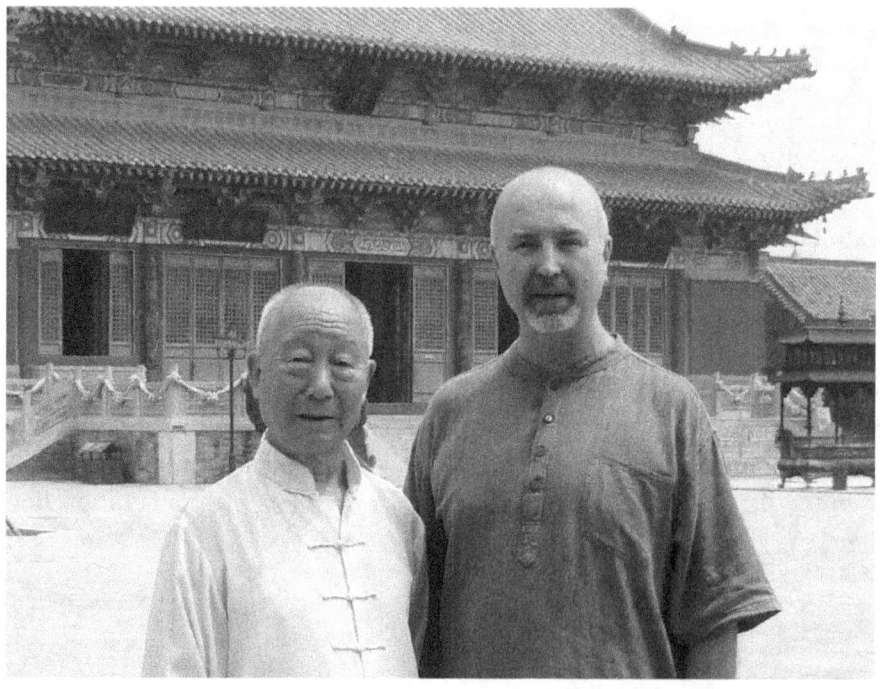

写在前面

西蒙·布劳先生是一位从事中外文化交流的学者，20多年来，遍访中国的名山大川，学习中国养生文化。并把传播中国传统养生文化作为一种终生职责。

2007年他访问武汉时习练了大雁气功。经人介绍结识了我。从此每年都来武汉认真刻苦的学习大雁气功。认为大雁气功是最好的养生术。他热爱大雁气功。

作为学生，他尊师重道，谦虚求教，勤奋学习。他这种精益求精的学习精神，使我很受感动！他学习了大雁气功前后64式基础功法，已习练三千遍以上。他精心刻苦的修炼，深得功中奥妙。并且在澳大利亚广泛传播大雁气功，队伍越来越壮大。

作为老师，他对教学言传身教，不厌其烦的细心教学，通俗易懂的讲解，使学生受益非浅。得到了学生们的爱戴。

他每年都带学生来中国深造，他带学生习练时，让我在一旁观察，纠正动作。这种方法教学在我的学生中也是少有的，应该来习练。他是一位优秀的大雁气功师。是我的入门第子。是大雁功在国外最好的29代传人。

为了更好的传播大雁功，依玖正、惟实的教学系列，西蒙根据活气功、教学体悟，写了一本英文版大雁功。并和我多次校正、讨示、定稿。这是一本依改宗师之宗、功法、动作准确、符合原貌、寓意丝毫没有个人成份的大雁功教材。是我所见到的英文版大雁功最惟宵的版本。望习功者之英阅读。

我祝贺西蒙大雁功英文版出版成功！

祝愿西蒙在海外宏扬、发展大雁功的成绩更加优异！

祝愿大雁功这神奇活译的功法在世界各地开花结果！越来越兴旺！

我们共同为大雁功为人类的健康作出应有的贡献！

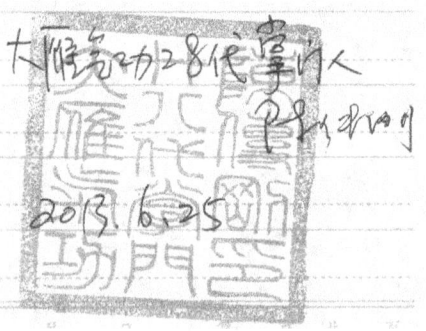

大雁气功28代掌门人
2013.6.25

About the Author: Simon Blow

A near fatal accident at the age of nineteen led Simon to investigate various methods of healing and rejuvenation, a path he has been following ever since. Simon is a Sydney-based (Australia) master teacher (Laoshi) of the ancient Chinese art of longevity and has been leading regular classes for beginning and continuing students since 1990.

Having travelled the world to learn and explore this ancient art, Simon has received extensive training and certification from many respected sources: Traditional lineage Grand Masters, Traditional Chinese Medical hospitals and Daoist monasteries in China, Buddhist monasteries in Australia, and Hindu ashrams in India. He has been given authority to share these techniques through his teachings and publications.

Simon has received extensive personal training in the Da Yan Wild Goose Qigong from the 28th generation lineage holder Grand Master, Chen Chuan Gang, and is an initinated student and 29th generation of this ancient healing art.

He received World Health Organisation certification in medical Qigong clinical practice from the Xiyuan Hospital in Beijing and is a Standing Council Member of the World Academic Society of Medical Qigong in Beijing. He has also been initiated into Dragon Gate Daoism and given the name of Xin Si, meaning 'genuine wisdom'.

Simon has spent quality time on many occasions at the Ramana Ashram in Southern India under the sacred mountain of Arunachala, following the self-realisation practices of Sri Ramana Maharishi.

His dedication, compassion and wisdom also make Simon a sought-after keynote speaker, workshop and retreat facilitator. By demand he has created a series of Book/DVD sets and guided meditation CDs. He also helped produce CDs for the Sunnatram Forest Monastery, the YWCA Encore program and a series of Meditation CDs for children and teenagers.

China holds a special place in Simon's heart. He has had the great fortune to travel to China on many occasions to study Qigong, attend international conferences, tour the sacred mountains and experience the rich culture of the Chinese people. Since 1999 he has been leading unique study tours to China so he could take people to the source and give them the opportunity to experience first-hand this ancient healing practice.

Romanisation of Chinese words

The Genuine Wisdom Centre uses the Pinyin romanisation system of Chinese to English. Pinyin is a name for the system used to transliterate Chinese words into the Roman alphabet. The use of Pinyin was first adopted in the 1950s by the Chinese government, and it became official in 1979 when it was endorsed by the People's Republic of China.

Pinyin is now standard in the People's Republic of China and in several world organisations, including the United Nations. Pinyin replaces the Wade-Giles and Yale systems.

Some common conversions:

Pinyin	Also spelled as	Pronunciation
Qi	Chi	Chee
Qigong	Chi Kung	Chee Kung
Tai Ji	Tai Chi	Tai Jee
Taijiquan	Tai Chi Chuan	Tai Jee Chuen
Gongfu	Kung Fu	Gong Foo
Dao	Tao	Dao
Daoism	Taoism	Daoism
Dao De Jing	Tao Teh Ching	Dao Teh Ching

The use of Chinese characters in this publication

Chinese writing has been a developing medium for thousands of years and is the oldest continuously used system of writing in the world. It's the foundation of many of the other Asian styles of writing, originating from simple pictures to complex brush strokes with many thousands of individual characters. Since the 1950s, traditional characters which numbered to the tens of thousands have been simplified to four or five thousand. Even though there are many different dialects spoken in China, including Mandarin and Cantonese, the characters remain the same and their written technique and meaning are taught in all schools across China. The computerised font used for Chinese characters which are used today and in this publication are simplified Chinese and some of the deeper meaning or essence from the ancient times has been lost in the translation from traditional to simplified characters.

A good example is the word 'Qi' as written in Pinyin or sometimes written as 'Chi', which is used to describe the energy of life or life-force energy.

氣 The traditional character for Qi shows a picture of a pot being heated on a fire or cooking of rice with steam smouldering from the top as a result of the cooking or the refining process of cultivating the internal energy.

气 The simplified character for Qi only shows the steam rising and is sometimes translated as air or breath, losing the deeper understanding of cultivation or refinement.

How to use this book

Da Yan Wild Goose Qigong is a very complex dynamic set of exercises. The book gives detailed instructions on how to perform the movements and provides additional theory and history to complement the practices. To view videos showing the shape of the movements
please visit out YouTube channel
www.youtube.com/simonblowqigong

It's important to learn from an experienced qualified teacher and to practise reguarly to master the movements yourself. Attending regular classes provides consistent practice and refinement and the energy of the group nurtures and supports everyone. It's important not to stray too far from the flock.

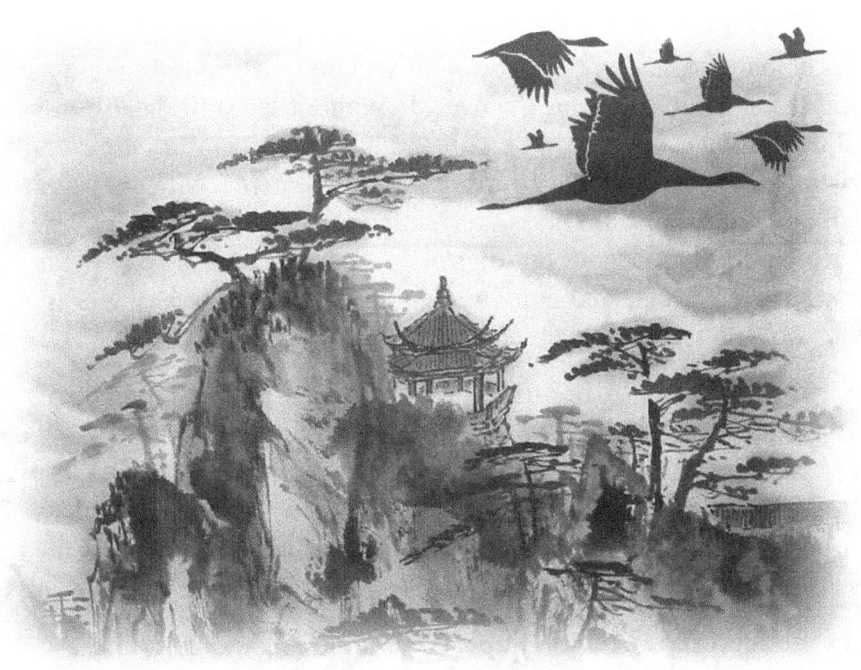

Chapter 1

Introduction

Da Yan - Wild Goose Qigong

The 1st 64 movements

Introduction

We as human beings have been on a constant search or quest to find meaning, happiness and fulfilment in our world. Without a strong healthy body and a calm emotional life, it can be very difficult to allow our true identity, our spirit or our consciousness to awaken and to merge with the divine. The mind, body and spirit are all equally important; they are collectively one or whole. All these aspects of our existence respond and can grow with regular maintenance, exercise and cultivation, allowing us to increase our quality of life and to fully appreciate the beauty of our world.

Sometimes we tend to be too focused on achieving external goals or on accumulating material possessions with the idea of becoming successful and happy. While it's important to be motivated, at an excessive or extreme level this can cause stress and anxiety and can deplete our quality of life. Maintaining a healthy life is finding balance and harmony within all the aspects of our world.

An important component of Chinese culture and Traditional Chinese Medicine (TCM) is the principle of 'Yang Sheng'. 'Yang' translates to 'taking care of', to 'nourish' or 'nurture' and 'Sheng' translates to 'birth' and 'vitality'. Together the words mean to 'nurture or nourish life', to 'foster a state of wellbeing by nurturing mind, body and spirit'. Yang Sheng is a manageable practice for all people, aimed at cultivating health and harmony through daily activities. The focus is on maintaining balance through an awareness of our connection with nature and our environment, our physical bodies and our spirit. Health preservation (instead of disease treatment) is an essential feature of TCM practice and is significantly different to Western medicine, which mainly focuses on disease and illness.

Many of the Yang Sheng principles are outlined in the book *Huangdi Neijing* or *The Yellow Emperor's Internal Canon of Chinese Medicine*, which dates back 2500 years. From my own experience of studying the Chinese healing arts and travelling to China on many occasions, my Chinese teachers and friends have been continuously educating me in a basic understanding of Yang Sheng: On why we eat certain foods and how the dishes are arranged and balanced with heating and cooling elements to balance Yin and Yang, how drinking warm green tea cleanses the fats from food and aids in our digestion, to remain calm and not waste our energy and to learn to sit quietly to cultivate the mind and nurture the spirit.

The study and practice of Qigong is the key element of Yang Sheng health cultivation. When we circulate Qi and clear stagnations within our meridians or energy system, this enables our Qi field or aura to increase, allowing us to achieve harmony in mind, body and spirit.

> *'Too much color, the eyes cannot enjoy.*
> *Too much noise, the ears cannot receive, and music cannot be heard or appreciated.*
> *Too complicated, too prepared, or too processed food causes the tongue to lose its taste.*
> *Too much rushing around, hunting and searching, maddens the mind.*
> *Too much interest in hard-to-obtain goods distorts one's behaviour.*
> *The wise one likes to maintain one's inner essence, and thus is not enslaved by sensory pleasure.*
> *Sensory pleasures and the outer search for material goods create burdens and cause one's life to become scattered.'*
> **Lao Tzu, Dao De Jing, Chapter 12**

Qigong

The word Qigong is made up of two Chinese characters, 'Qi' and 'Gong'. 'Qi' (Chi) translates to the 'energy of life', the vital energy which flows through the network of meridians in the body and connects with the energy or Qi of the universe. In Japan and Korea it's known as 'Ki' and if studying Yoga the term 'Prana' is used. Most cultures have a similar terminology for life energy. 'Gong' (Kung) is a term which translates to 'work, mastery, skill and training'. The two words therefore translate to 'energy work', 'working with the energy of life' or 'mastering the energy of life'.

The practices of Qigong date back many thousands of years and the underlining principles and concepts are intertwined with Chinese culture. An older term for these energetic practices that has been used since ancient times is 'Daoyin', which translates to 'guiding exercises'. The word Qigong has only been used since the 1950s as a way of classifying all the Qi or energy techniques. It can be categorised into three separate sections; Martial/Sports Qigong, Medical/Healing Qigong and Spiritual/Meditation Qigong and within these sections there are hundreds or even thousands of sub-categories. Qigong is one of the great treasures of Chinese culture and an integral component of Chinese medical health systems. The understanding and cultivation of Qi is one of the underlying principles of Daoist, Buddhist and Confucius practices, as well as the martial arts. The art of Qigong consists primarily of meditation, relaxation, physical movement, mind-body integration and breathing exercises. There are thousands of different styles and systems practised: done standing, moving, walking, sitting or lying down. Taijiquan or Tai Chi is one more popular style.

From ancient times, Qigong was developed as a way of helping improve people's quality of life. When the mind and body come into a state of balance, stress is reduced and there is an increase in health and longevity. This allows us to become naturally in harmony with our environment and the universe. Many of the ancient Qigong styles reflect this state of harmony and balance by adapting the natural flowing movements of birds, animals and serpents.

Da Yan Wild Goose

'Da Yan' translates to 'great bird' and is an ancient Qigong practice originating from the Kunlun School of Daoism in the Jin Dynasty about 1700 years ago. Legend tells that Daoist masters from the sacred Kunlun Mountains, in the northern Himalayan area in south-west China, would observe the migrating geese which descended in this area each year. They would mimic the movements of these great birds and together with their understanding of Traditional Chinese Medicine and Daoist principles, developed the Da Yan Wild Goose Qigong system.

Its healing and spiritual legacy was passed down through many generations, however Da Yan Qigong was withheld from the general public until 1978. Then 27th generation lineage holder Grand Master Yang Mei Jung (1895-2002) decided to teach this ancient Qigong practice and share its healing benefits to improve the quality of life of all people. Da Yan Qigong is a complete Qigong healing system. Practitioners and Qigong enthusiasts from all over China and other countries worldwide have come to learn from Grand Master Yang Mei Jung.

The foundation of the Da Yan Qigong system is the 1st and 2nd 64 movement sets; the movements representing the flight of wild geese. There are slow graceful movements and strong quick movements designed to release stale Qi and to gather fresh Qi, helping to restore balance and stimulate the entire energy system of the body. The number sixty-four is a very auspicious combination of numbers in Chinese philosophy and is related to the sixty-four hexagrams of the *Yijing (I Ching)*, or *Book of Changes.*

The 1st 64 movement set deals primary with the 'postnatal body'. In traditional Daoist understanding, this refers to 'after heaven', relating to the energy that one gathers after birth, especially from breathing and food. This first set is very important as it addresses injuries and illness that we have acquired during this lifetime. It works on the twelve primary organ meridians, the collaterals and emphasises the Ren, Du, Chong and Dai channels of the body. In the 1st 64 movement set, the movements represent the daily activities of the goose as it exercises its body in its local environment and gains essence from the food, water and air.

The 2nd 64 movement set deals primarily with the 'prenatal body'. This refers to 'before heaven', relating to the energy we gather from the universe and from one's ancestors, addressing problems that have been genetically inherited. Having dredged the channels in the first form, the 2nd 64 movement set is designed to clear the channels to absorb fresh Qi, expel stale Qi and to restore organ balance. The twisting, stretching, bending and pressing movements produce stronger Qi fields and intensify the circulation of the eight extraordinary channels. In the 2nd 64 movement set the goose is embarking on a great journey and flies out from this world to the edge of the Milky Way, to pick the herbs or gather the prenatal Qi from the core of the universe. It then flies back to this world to share this healing energy with humanity.

When we come into this world we are born with two internal batteries. One is filled with the essence, energy and spirit from the universe and our ancestors, or what is inherited by us. The second is the battery that we make ourselves, from our own endeavours and the connections that we make in this world. We become our own internal alchemist cultivating our essence, energy and spirit and with the correct knowledge, discipline the practice, we are able to increase and improve our quality of life.

All the Chinese healing exercises help aid in our development and nurture mind, body and spirit. The Da Yan Wild Goose Qigong is a very powerful exercise and throughout history has proven to improve longevity. My teacher Grand Master Chen Chuan Gang is ninety years of age and he is still very active, teaching classes each day as well as travelling to other parts of China promoting his family's skill. His mother, Grand Master Yang Mei Jung, passed away at the age of one hundred and six and she was also very active right up to the time of her passing, teaching and sharing all that she knew so others could benefit.

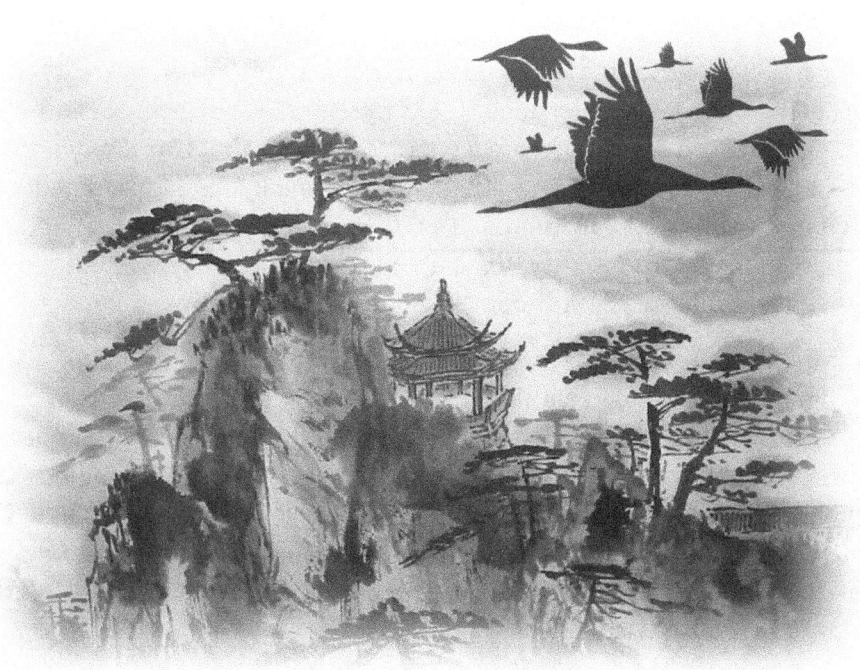

Chapter 2

The Details - how does it work?

Da Yan - Wild Goose Qigong

The 1st 64 movements

The Details - how does it work?

When we start our journey into the Chinese healing arts there are many new ideas and concepts to understand. It's different to the exercises that many of us may have been taught when we were younger or that is promoted through gyms and other sporting activities. They're even quite different to yoga which are a very popular mind and body exercise. The key to the practices are relaxation and tranquillity; to be able to move the body without too much physical or mental tension. It does take practice, a lot of practice.

It's important to grasp the basic theory and the philosophy of the Chinese healing arts. Otherwise without this understanding, these ancient energy cultivation practices can become a slow motion dance or gentle exercises. To understand the theory is important, but the practice is more important. It's only through constant practice over many years that the concepts and theory become intertwined with our thought processes and it becomes natural. When this happens, the true benefits of the Chinese healing arts can be realised.

Da Yan Wild Goose Qigong is a very complex set of movements and it does take time to master. The Chinese have a term for this Gong Fu (Kung Fu); 'Gong' means 'work, skill or cultivation' and 'Fu' means 'time'. Together these two words translate to 'taking the time to cultivate a skill'. Sometimes the longer it takes, the better the result will be. This two book series on the 1st 64 movement and 2nd 64 movement sets are designed as instruction aids, allowing you to gain a clear understanding of how to perform each movement, how it works and its history and philosophy. It also features inspiring stories from those who have been practising Da Yan Qigong and the Chinese healing arts to help increase their quality of life. The 1st 64 movement set is the most important as it establishes a solid foundation; the movements repetitively purge the meridians or energy channels, allowing our mind and body to find harmony and to rebalance. It's only when we have mastered the movements and details of the 1st 64 movement set that we can move on to the 2nd 64 movement set. A classic Chinese saying says, 'To practise a thousand times and the effects will show.' The first level of training is to learn the form, the shape of each posture and the sequence of movements. The second level is to learn all the details, which include the major meridians' acupoints. The third level of training is to learn the Qi or energy flow. If the movement is not correct, clear and accurate, the details will not be correct and then the Qi flow will not be correct.

The three levels of training in the Da Yan Wild Goose Qigong system:

1.   **Practising the physical movements**
2.   **Practising the details**
3.   **Practising the Qi or energy flow**

Wu Ji 無 極 and Tai Ji 太 極

According to Chinese philosophy, before heaven or before creation was the state of Wu Ji. It is also known as prenatal in Traditional Chinese Medicine (TCM) literature. The primordial universe was in a state of nothingness, emptiness, the void, before creation as we know it; before the big bang. After the big bang came the after heaven or postnatal state of the universe; this is what the Chinese call 'Tai Ji' also popularly written as 'Tai Chi'. 'Something came from nothing' as the classics say, the two opposing forces of Yin and Yang created the after heaven universe. This can be seen in the Tai Ji symbol which comprises two opposing forces that balance or complement each other. Without one the other would not exist. Yang energy is expressed in qualities such as up, external, male, hot and bright. Yin energy resides in the opposing characteristics such as down, internal, female, cold and dark.

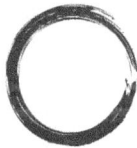

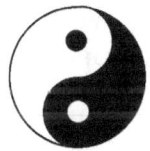

Wu Ji Symbol   Tai Ji Symbol

Seven Stars Constellation

There are many combinations of movements within the Da Yan Wild Goose Qigong system and many of these are repeated seven times. This relates to the seven stars of the big dipper which are clearly visible in the evening sky.

The ancient Chinese said that those seven stars represent the Emperor's carriage (the vehicle of God's will), rotating around the centre of the universe. It governs the Four Directions, and divides Yin from Yang. It determines the Four Seasons and balances the Five Elements According to modern astronomy the Earth's rotation axis points toward this area, which is the north pole of what is called the sphere of the sky or the celestial sphere. It is the celestial sphere that rotates or appears to rotate around an axis defined by the Chinese constellation of the Emperor's Chariot.

At the Hubei Provincial Museum in Wuhan, China is the Tomb of Marquis Yi of Zeng, which was accidently discovered in 1977 and has been dated to

500 BC. One of the artefacts found was a wooden travelling box or suitcase with the seven stars clearly inlayed on the top, a bit like an address to send the luggage to.

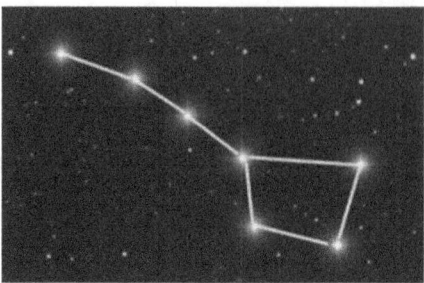

Seven Stars Constellation

Dao 道 or Tao translates to 'the way' or 'path'. It's not a religion but a way of connecting and harmonising with nature. Its origins are in ancient Chinese culture dating back over 5000 years. Lao Tzu, a historical figure from 500 BC, was the first great master to write about his understanding of the nature of the Dao. His book, the *Dao De Jing*, now forms the basis of most Daoist thought. Some of the other healing arts originating from Daoist tradition include acupuncture, Chinese herbal medicine, Qigong, Taijiquan, Feng Shui and Chinese therapeutic massage.

The Three Treasures is one of the foundation principles of Daoism and TCM. It's a way of understanding how we as human beings grow internally and connect with our environment and universe. Unfortunately if our internal energy system is not functioning correctly this natural process will suffer and we will not fully experience the beauty of life as we should.

Jing 精 or Essence refers to all refined, subtle, and nutritious substances and is the material basis of the human body. We receive Jing in two ways, from what we are born with (prenatal), from our family heritage; a bit like energetic DNA. We also receive essence from the fresh food, water and air that nourishes our body in the present world (postnatal). It is important to protect the Jing that has been given to us. Illness, stress and an unhealthy lifestyle will waste this precious energy

Qi 氣 or Energy can be translated as 'natural energy', 'life force' or 'energy flow' and refers to the refined subtle essences. According to TCM, Qi controls the functional activities of the organs in the body. The Qi inherent in the prenatal state is called 'original' or 'Yuan Qi' and the Qi obtained from breathing and diet is called 'acquired' Qi. There are many different types of Qi, depending on distribution, locations and its function. There are three main aspects of Qi; 'Heaven Qi' is the Yang energy that we absorb from the universe, 'Earth Qi' is the Yin energy that we receive from this world and 'Human Qi' is the interrelationship between the energies of heaven and earth, the harmony between Yang and Yin.

Shen 神 or Spirit is the governor of life activities according to TCM theory. Shen represents the active nature of our being, including our presence, consciousness, vitality, mental functions and spiritual activities. Through the Shen we are able to project ourselves and connect with the energies of the universe and the divine. The prenatal Shen refers to the light from our original nature before birth and the postnatal Shen is sometimes called the 'acquired' or 'mind of desires' spirit.

Cultivating the Three Treasures - Essence, Energy and Spirit
The Yellow Emperor's Internal Classic says, 'The original substances of life is called Jing (Essence); the combined Yin and Yang essence is called spirit (Shen).' These internal cultivation practices are divided into four stages of cultivation: refining Jing (Essence) and converting it into Qi (Energy), refining Qi to nourish the Shen (Spirit), refining Shen to return to nothingness and refining nothingness to integrate into Dao. The stage of refining essence to convert it into Qi is also termed the 'Small Heavenly Orbit Circulation'.

Dan Tian 丹田 translates to 'the cauldron where elixir is refined'. There are three Dan Tians or energy centres in the body according to Daoist and TCM understanding. They are like a storehouse or reservoir where the cultivated internal energy is stored for later use. The lower Dan Tian is situated just below the navel and is the foundation for standing, breathing and body awareness; it is where essence or Jing is refined into Qi. The middle Dan Tian is at the level of the heart and is associated with respiration and the health of the internal organs; this is also where the spirit or Shen resides and is where Qi is refined into Shen. The upper Dan Tian is between the eyebrows and is where Shen is refined into nothingness.

Traditional Chinese Medicine
An important principle underlying Traditional Chinese Medicine (TCM) is the understanding of the balance and harmony between human beings and our environment. Daoism and TCM view the human being as a micro (internal) representation of our macro (external) environment. It is based on the concept that the human body is a small universe with a set of complete and sophisticated interconnected systems, and that those systems usually work in

balance and with the forces of nature to maintain the healthy function of the human body. TCM seeks to heal the root causes of dysfunction or disease and has been practised for over 5000 years, making it one of the oldest and most widely used systems of medicine in the world.

In this ancient vision of the body, the internal organs function differently from the way they are understood to function in Western medicine. Unlike the Western medical model which divides the physical body into anatomical structures, the Chinese model is more concerned with function. Thus, the TCM heart is not a specific piece of flesh, but an aspect of function related to consciousness, mental vitality and unclouded thinking.

Each solid organ (Yin) has a corresponding flowing organ (Yang). TCM understands that everything is composed of two complementary energies; one energy is Yin and the other is Yang. They are never separate; one cannot exist without the other. This relationship is reflected in the black and white Yin/Yang symbol. No matter how you try to divide this circle in half, each section will always contain both energies.

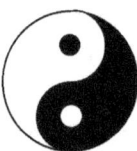

The organs also correspond to the Five Elements, relating to different seasons, directions, colours and emotions. The belief that the human body is a microcosm of the universal macrocosm means that humans must follow the laws of the universe to achieve harmony and total health. The Yin/Yang and Five Element theories are observations and descriptions of universal law, not concepts created by man. These essential theories form the basis of TCM and are used today to understand, diagnose and treat health problems. The network of relationships is complex and scholars study and meditate for many years to fully understand these connections between the internal and the external world.

	EARTH 土	METAL 金	WATER 木	WOOD 水	FIRE 火
Organ (Yin)	Spleen	Lungs	Kidneys	Liver	Heart
Organ (Yang)	Stomach	Large Intestine	Urinary Bladder	Gall Bladder	Small Intestine
Season	Late summer	Autumn	Winter	Spring	Summer
Plant Part	Fruit	Compost	Seed	Shoot	Flower
Function	Harvest	Death	Storing	Sprouting	Blossoming
Emotion	Worry	Grief	Fear	Anger	Joy/Excitement
Colour	Yellow	White	Deep Blue/Black	Green	Red
Type of Qi	Dampness	Dryness	Cold	Wind	Heat
Direction	Centre	West	North	East	South
Senses	Skin, touch	Nose, smell	Ears, hearing	Eyes, sight	Tongue, taste

Meridians

While Western medicine recognises only three circulatory networks in the human body the nervous system, the lymphatic system and the blood vessels, TCM includes a fourth system: the energy network of meridians. Meridians are pathways or channels which transport Qi through the whole body, ensuring the tissues and organs are supplied with fluids and nutrients. They are all interconnected and form a network to connect the internal organs to external parts of the body.

Meridian lines or energy channels cannot be seen or felt like other systems in the body such as the circulatory or nervous system. When a person is in good (balanced) health, their meridian lines will be open and clear of blockages. Qi can then flow smoothly.

These meridian lines can be associated with the functioning of the body's internal organs. The health of an organ is affected by the corresponding meridian and has a direct impact on the strength and energy of the meridian. If these organs function abnormally, the energy will stagnate in the meridians and cause illness. To return to good health the blockage must be released and the flow of energy normalised.

The Twelve Organ Meridians or Energy Channels
(see back of book for full diagrams)

No 1. Lung Meridian 肺 经 (Yin) Nurturing. The main purpose of the lungs is respiration. According to TCM, the lungs are in charge of the Qi of the whole body.

No 2. Large Intestine Meridian 大 肠 经 (Yang) Dispersing. The large intestine's function is to pass and eliminate waste.

No 3. Spleen Meridian 脾 经 (Yin) Nurturing. The spleen aids in the digestive system and in TCM the essence received from food and water is distributed to all parts of the body.

No 4. Stomach Meridian 胃 经 (Yang) Dispersing. The stomach also aids in absorption and digestion; the stomach likes to be moist, allowing the Qi to descend.

No 5. Liver Meridian 肝 经 (Yin) Nurturing. The liver helps regulate and smooth the flow of blood and Qi. It promotes digestion and absorption as well as keeping Qi and blood moving normally

No 6. Gall Bladder Meridian 胆 经 (Yang) Dispersing. The gall bladder receives the bile that is made and secreted by the liver.

No 7. Kidney Meridian 肾 经 (Yin) Nurturing. In TCM, the kidneys store the essence that is received from food and air and is released when the other organs require it. They are similar to batteries of the body.

No 8. Bladder Meridian 膀 胱 经 (Yang) Dispersing. After the kidneys have cleansed the fluids in the body, the clean fluids are retained and the waste is stored and excreted by the bladder.

No 9. Heart Meridian 心 经 (Yin) Nurturing. The heart is the 'Emperor of the body' according to ancient TCM texts. It helps control the function of the whole body.

No 10. Small Intestine Meridian 小 肠 经 (Yang) Dispersing. The small intestine receives, transforms and absorbs the solids and fluids, helping to separate the waste from any useful parts.

No 11. Pericardium Meridian 心 包 经 (Yin) Nurturing. The pericardium also relates to the functions of the heart.

No 12. Triple Heater (Sanjao) Meridian 三 焦 经 (Yang) Dispersing. The triple heater is a passage in which solids and fluids are heated and pass through the body.

The Meridian Cycle

Meridians are classified as Yin or Yang depending on which way they flow on the surface of the body. Yang energy flows from the sun, and Yang meridians run from the fingers to the face or from the face to the feet. Yin energy flows from the earth, flows from the feet to the torso and from the torso along the inside of the arms to the fingertips. Since the meridian flow is continuous and unbroken, the energy flows in one direction and from one meridian to another in a well determined order. Since there is no beginning or end to this flow, the order can be represented as a wheel. The flow around the wheel follows the meridian lines on the body in this order:

- From torso to fingertip (along inside of arm – Yin)
- From fingertip to face (along outside/back of arm – Yang)
- From face to feet (along outside of leg – Yang)
- From feet to torso (along inside of the leg – Yin)

The Eight Extra Ordinary Channels

These meridians or energy channels crisscross the regular organ meridians and perform the function of strengthening the ties between the channels and regulating the Qi and blood inside the twelve regular meridians.
(See back of book for full diagrams)

No 1. The Du Channel 督 脉. The word Du translates to 'a general superintendent'. This channel governs all of the Yang channels. It's also known as the 'sea' of all Yang channels.

No 2. The Ren Channel 任 脉. The word Ren in Chinese means 'take charge' and this channel governs all the Yin channels.

No 3. The Chong Channel 冲 脉. It is also called the 'sea of the twelve channels' and regulates the circulation of Qi and blood by communicating with the main organ channels.

No 4. The Dai Channel 带 脉 (Girdle Vessel). This runs around the waist like a belt and is usually described as 'binding' all the channels.

No 5. The Yin Qiao Channel 阴 跷 脉. This controls the Yin channels of the left and right sides of the body as well as nourishing the eyes and the motion of the lower limbs.

No 6. The Yang Qiao Channel 阳 跷 脉. 'Qiao' means 'nimble' in Chinese. It controls the Yang channels of the left and right sides of the whole body.

No 7. The Yin Wei Channel 阴 维 脉. 'Wei' translates to 'maintain' and 'communicate'. The Wei Yin ties together the Yin channels, connecting and regulating all of them.

No 8. The Yang Wei Channel 阳 维 脉. This ties together the Yang channels, connecting and regulating them all.

Meridian Acupoints
Along the meridian channels are specific locations which can be stimulated either with pressure, needles or by applying heat using modern lasers, or the ancient method of burning herbs as in moxibustion. Qigong also uses these acupoints to stimulate the meridian system and balance Yin and Yang. The Qigong acupoints are larger in scope and correspond to regions, whereas the acupoints used in acupuncture and moxibustion have a narrower scope, corresponding to points.

The Small and Large Heavenly Orbit
The Heavenly Orbit, also known as the 'Micro Cosmic Orbit' refers to the flow of energy or Qi in and around the body along the extraordinary channels. Yang energy rises up the back along the Du channel, nourishing the Yang organ meridians and Yin energy descends down the front along the Ren channel, nourishing all the Yin organ meridians. The Small Orbit refers to the flow of Qi around the torso from the base of the body (Hui Yin), to the top of the head (Bai Hui). The Large Orbit follows the same path and branches out from the base of the body at the Hui Yin, down the outside of the legs to the feet and onto the tip of the toes, up the inside of the legs to the Hui Yin at the base of the body, then the circle continues up the back to the base of the skull (Yu Zhen), down the inside of the arms to the fingertips, then back up the outside of the arms to the Yu Shen, then to the base of the skull, continuing the orbit.

The TCM and Daoist understanding of the energy channels can differ. In TCM the Ren channel flows from the lower abdomen up to the jaw, whereas in Daoist Qigong, the Ren channel flows down from the jaw to the lower abdomen. The Qigong theory is that this flow of energy is similar to the flow of water; continuously flowing, permeating and stimulating the meridian system and rebalancing the energy system of the body. It enables the blood to flow smoothly and the organs to function correctly, secreting different fluids and chemicals and allowing the body to restore natural harmony. It also helps calm the emotions as the mind is not distracted by the imbalances it detects. It resembles a large living Tai Ji symbol, constantly flowing around the body balancing and harmonising Yin and Yang. This energy system works on many levels. Every cell of the body is similar to a tiny moving Tai Ji. When our Qi or energy is weak, this orbit doesn't flow very smoothly, affecting our quality of life.

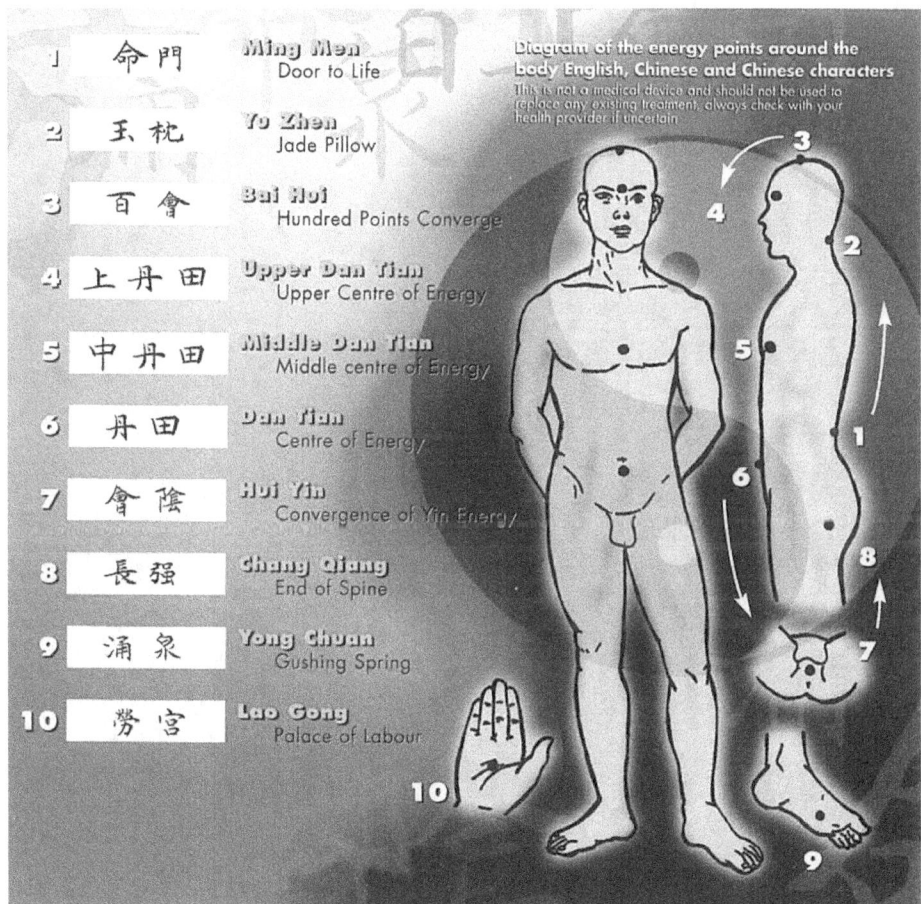

		Chinese	English	Meaning
1	命門	Ming Men	Door to Life
2	玉枕	Yo Zhen	Jade Pillow
3	百會	Bai Hui	Hundred Points Converge
4	上丹田	Upper Dan Tian	Upper Centre of Energy
5	中丹田	Middle Dan Tian	Middle centre of Energy
6	丹田	Dan Tian	Centre of Energy
7	會陰	Hui Yin	Convergence of Yin Energy
8	長強	Chang Qiang	End of Spine
9	涌泉	Yong Chuan	Gushing Spring
10	勞宮	Lao Gong	Palace of Labour

Diagram of the energy points around the body English, Chinese and Chinese characters

This is not a medical device and should not be used to replace any existing treatment, always check with your health provider if uncertain

The Five Steps for Qi Training in the Da Yan Qigong System

1. Qi circulation around the small and large Heavenly Orbit
2. Qi circulation around the Five Organs
3. Qi circulation in and around in a spiral direction
4. Flow of Qi to be gentle and smooth
5. Utilising, absorbing, gathering, dispersing and emitting Qi.

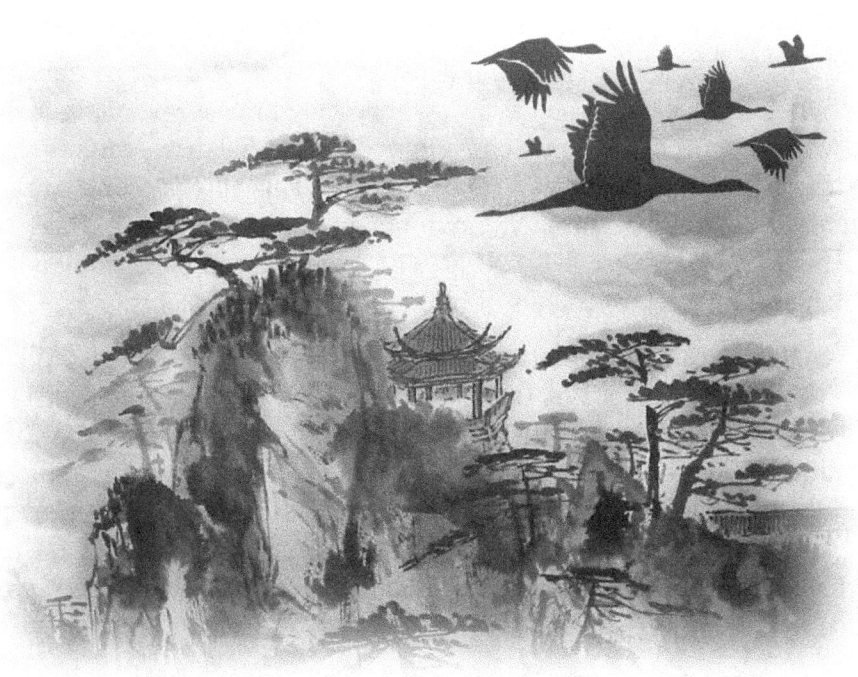

Chapter 3

The History

Da Yan - Wild Goose Qigong
The 1st 64 movements

The History

The Chinese culture has a long proud history of over 5000 years. From ancient times, Qigong was developed as a way of helping improve people's quality of life. When the mind and body come into a state of balance, stress is reduced and there is an increase in health and longevity. This allows people to become naturally in harmony with their environment and the universe. Many of the ancient Qigong styles reflect this state of harmony and balance by adapting the natural flowing movements of birds, animals and serpents.

Da Yan translates to 'great bird' and is an ancient Qigong practice originating from the Kunlun School of Daoism in the Jin Dynasty (265-420). Legend tells that Daoist masters from the sacred Kunlun Mountains, in the northern Himalayan area in south-west China, would observe the migrating geese which descended in this area each year. They would mimic the movements of these great birds and together with their understanding of Traditional Chinese Medicine and Daoist principles, developed the Da Yan Wild Goose Qigong system.

Dao An was the name of the Buddhist monk who is accredited as the spiritual father of the Da Yan Wild Goose Qigong. He was brought up in a Daoist family during the Jin Dynasty (265-420). Stories of Dao An tell that he was born with a few physical deformities. At a young age his family thought it best that he spend his life in a Buddhist monastery away from the hurtful taunts of other children. Dao An proved to be highly intelligent and of a strong moral character. He rose through the ranks of the monastery and was accredited with translating many of the sacred Sanskrit Buddhist texts into Chinese. Through his deep knowledge of the spiritual and physical worlds, Dao An made a major contribution to the development of the Da Yan Wild Goose Qigong system.

Its healing and spiritual legacy was passed down through many generations, however Da Yan Wild Goose Qigong was withheld from the general public until 1978. Then 27th generation lineage holder Grand Master Yang Mei Jung (1895-2002) decided to teach this ancient Qigong practice and share its healing benefits to improve the quality of life of all people. Yang Mei Jung was from a traditional Daoist family and from the age of thirteen was personally taught in secret by her Grandfather Yang De Shan, the 26th generation lineage holder. A young Yang Mei Jung was told by her grandfather that she was the next lineage holder and that he would pass on to her all the history, theory and knowledge of this ancient healing system. These secret cultivation practices were to be kept to herself so she could develop, understand and nurture this ancient wisdom. She was not allowed to pass on this information to anyone until she reached the age of seventy.

During the Cultural Revolution (1966-1976), Qigong and other healing and spiritual practices were banned. This period in Chinese history affected the country socially and economically for many years. When reforms were lifted in 1976, the then leader Deng Xiao Ping famously said 'let everyone dance'. From that time people started to take to the streets and parks to once again practise all the different types of Chinese healing exercises. In 1978 at the age of eighty-three, Yang Mei Jung observed this new freedom of expression, but she didn't like a lot of the Qigong that she saw and the claims that some people were making. Now was the time for Grand Master Yang Mei Jung, the 27th generation lineage holder of the Da Yan Wild Goose Qigong, to share this ancient healing practice. Being a lady in her eighties and of smaller stature, under five foot (150cm), she had an amazingly strong presence and energy. She started teaching in a park in Beijing and soon the word spread. Practitioners and Qigong enthusiasts from all over China and other countries worldwide came to learn from Grand Master Yang Mei Jung.

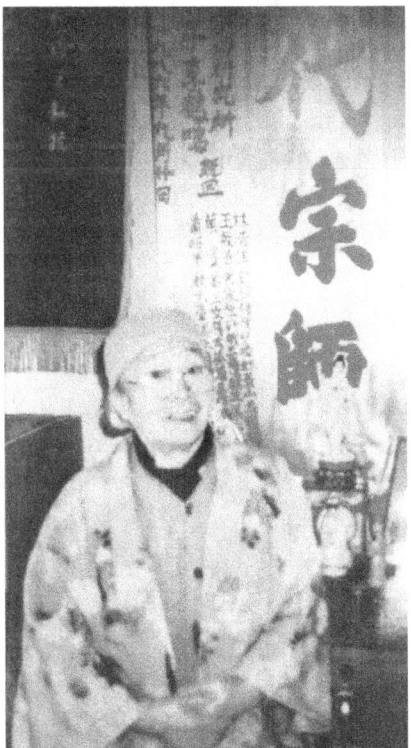 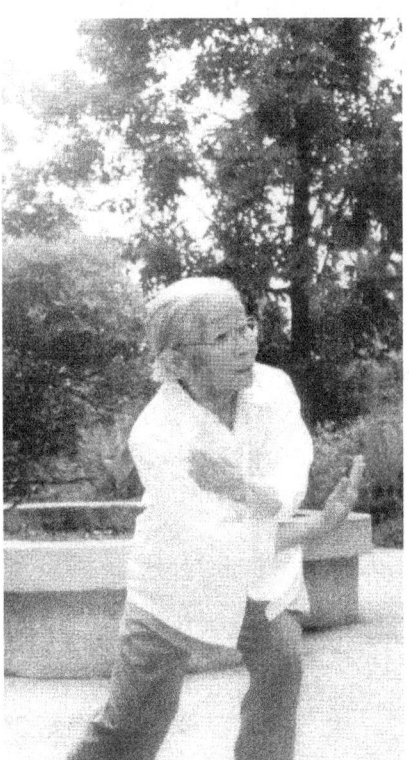

Grand Master Yang Mei Jung

Grand Master Yang Mei Jung passed away in 2002 at the age of one hundred and six. In 2012 on the tenth anniversary of her passing, her eldest son Chen Chaun Gang and 28th generation lineage holder, wrote the following memories of his mother. The original article has been translated from Chinese characters into English by Zhang Jing and briefly edited by myself and Master Chen. The family has given me permission to share this information so all can benefit and be inspired to learn and continue practising Da Yan Wild Goose Qigong.

Memories of my mother

'My mother is a kind-hearted woman. During my life, I wasn't living with mother very long. But I can never forget the unbelievable hardship and difficulty mother lived through to bring us children up. Her loving expressions on the face often appear in my mind; especially her determination to lead me into Qigong training with all her efforts by removing those obstacles and teaching me personally her own ways makes me feel heart-touching. Although she has been away from us for ten years, her familiar sound and features, her Daoist power and influence never diminish. Whenever I think of the every bit of treasure mother gave me I easily get moved and excited.

'Mother's miracle power was not known for a long time. I didn't know anything about it when I was a child. I only remember that we used to go with mother to the temples and the mountain shrines to pray and burn incense. Mother said, "These are Daoist blessings, there are many different kinds and they are all good for self-protection. You can try these in future to protect yourself." This might be my earliest knowledge for Qigong.

'The Second World War broke out. Like most people in China, my family fled home on an evacuation journey. All family members separated on the way. My father and two brothers died one after another; my mother and sister went on their own. I left mother, trying to make a living by myself. In 1942, I met mother in Han Dan, He Bei province. I was young then, I didn't even ask mum where came from and how she was living by herself. Later on I joined the Chinese Army and went to the frontline. I lost contact with mother again, I couldn't find her even after new China was born in 1949. This separation lasted for thirty-six years.

'In 1970s, I got news that mother was living in Beijing. I sent my children and friends to Beijing many times looking for her. But none of these attempts were successful. Eventually one of my friends Jin Yulan was able to meet mother in Beijing in 1979. Knowing I was looking for her, mother had a long talk with Jin Yulan, and demonstrated her some Qigong skills. Mother asked Jin Yulan to tell me that she was well and she wanted to see me soon. Finally we got in contact again.

'My formal training in Da Yan Gong began in 1980 when I met mother for the first time after thirty-six years. She was performing at a Qigong conference. She looked in high spirit that day with big voice. We were all in tears when we met. Her first words were, "I know you are still alive, I am looking after you, and I am protecting you. See this white porcelain jar under the bed? I moved the house many times, but the jar never got damaged. I know you are still alive and will come to look for me."

'In mother's house in Nan Mo Fang in Beijing, I had access to Qigong. Mother was proud showing some of her pictures taken with famous people and a slogan hanging on the wall saying, 'Qigong is science'. She said, "Probably you don't believe in Qigong but I do. Qigong is science. Let me send you some Qi to feel it." She asked me to put out my hand two meters away from her and she started twisting a piece of match that was pointing at my hand. I suddenly felt hot and numb all over my back like bugs crawling! Mother said, "Feel it? Believe it? This is Qigong." With this Kun Lun finger, mother led me through the Wild Goose gate.

'During my time with mother in Beijing this trip, I learned first 64 movements and basic meditation from her. She taught me both postures and theory. She said, "Even the best style of training, if you don't practice enough, it won't do you any good. You can remember movements by repeating them many times, but for theory you have to understand by using the heart." Since I returned home from this trip, I started to practise Wild Goose. I wasn't retired then, I had to find any time day and night available for the training, early morning, and late evening sometimes I practised at midnight. I made much progress for the benefit. All my friends noticed that I got Qi.

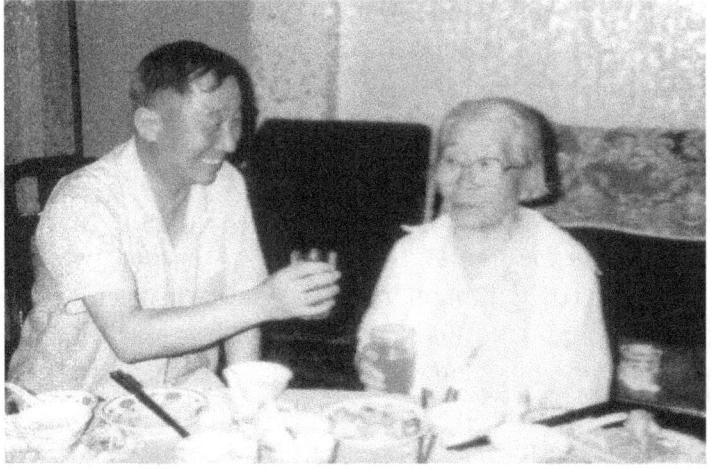

Grand Master Chen and Grand Master Yang Mei Jung - 1988

'From 1980-1984 I went to Beijing many times to learn the second 64 and some other secret forms. I also travelled with mother to Shanghai and Tianjin for Qigong conferences. Mother said, "Qigong comes from people; it has to serve the people for their health benefit. The Da Yan Wild Goose is the treasure of China so am I?" She wanted me to inherit it. She said, "You have to carry it on." One time we were practising together, I couldn't follow the others. I was looking around, trying to pick the right movements. Mother saw this, she gave me a slap on the face and said, "When we were students, we had to learn every movement by no more than three times that we were taught. I have made it clear many times, why haven't you got it? You must use your heart while getting rid of all other things to reach the state of nothingness. What is nothingness? It is between there and not there. This is the genuine training I teach. You must have faith in it." Afterwards I tried to figure out what she said about nothingness. You aim for nothing but you gain for everything. This is the miracle of nothingness.

'Another time when mother finished meditation, she asked us to sit around her to feel the Qi. I put out my hand, I felt strong Qi moving around her body in different directions. I realised this was the Qi of the orbit, different way of Qi moving in the orbit. Sometimes she asked us to do meditation at midnight, just watching and focusing 'the internal light'. During a teaching journey my Daoist brother Feng and I went with mother; several journalists came and asked mother questions. They wanted healing experiences from mother. Mother said, "These two students are very good with Qi now. Let them check up your health." I stood there still and wasn't sure if I was able to do the healing. Mother saw this and said, "Go." Immediately I felt full of Qi all over my body. Only after a few minutes the person sitting in front of me was sweating. He kept saying, "Good. Good." I knew this was the power transferred from mother. Only you have practised enough, you will be able to receive this external Qi and use it. My potential Qi for healing was triggered off by mother this time.

'As mother says, Wild Goose Qigong is a miracle training. It can be simple, can be complicated. It is broad and infinite. The training relies on practice. The theory is within the training. You do for everything while you do for nothing. Once you are led through inside the gate by master, your own efforts become the most important. Wild Goose emphasises practice not words. You will get benefit from your long time practice. This is the way mother used to teach me. The Wild Goose is based on the balance of hard power and soft power. The soft creates the hard. The weak creates the strong. Nothing creates something. If you overplay the hard, then too stiff, you won't get nothingness.

'From 1984-1990 I travelled with mother to different provinces to teach and run classes. During these periods of time, I noticed mother was trying to teach and pass her knowledge any time of the day. Sometimes I could feel the connection of Qi with mother. I learned some forms with both words and movements, also some forms only with words but no movements. For example one form only with these words, 'Dao creates one, I obtain one.' It means by saying these words you get the connection of Qi from the universe then you will be able to receive the Qi from both heaven and earth. High level Qigong training also requires the connection, perception and morality involved. Without these you won't get very high. Some of mother's students didn't have these qualities, instead they were selfish and they wanted the benefit of training only for themselves. Once they left mother, all they got from mother disappeared.

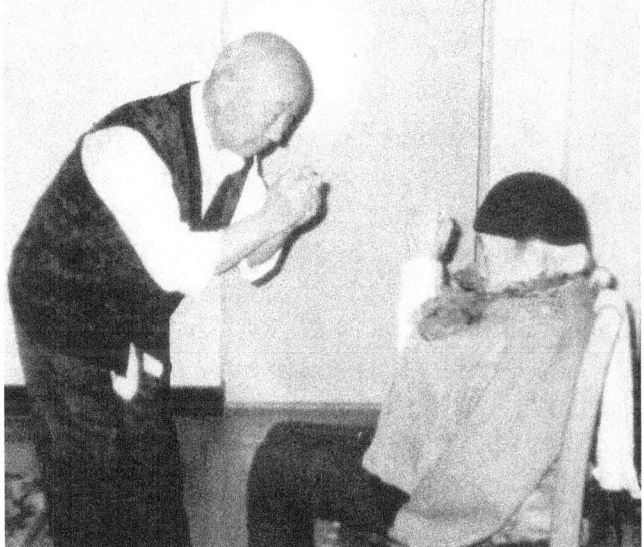

Grand Master Chen and Grand Master Yang Mei Jung - 1998

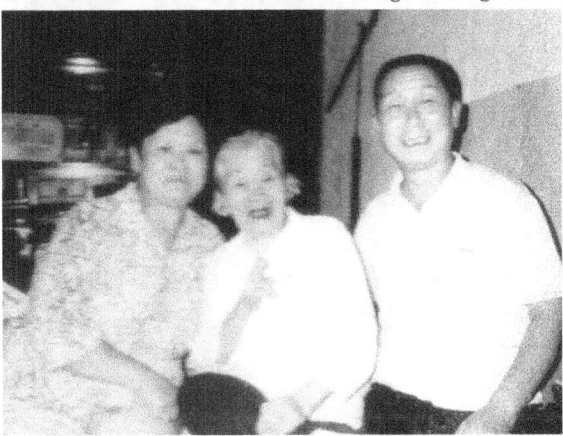

Madam Chen, Grand Master Yang Mei Jung and Grand Master Chen - 1993

'Mother used to tell me, "Given power is from masters. It is an important support. Chanting, leading meditation, touching students head are all considered given power, helping the students have stronger Qi. But the students have to make this power become their own so you could keep it long." Training for Dao requires the cultivation of heart. If you want to achieve Dao, you have to cultivate your internal world and that moral standard is important part of it. Benevolence, intelligence, loyalty, diligence, dignity are all the qualities you must have. This is the training for both life and spirit. Once I was talking with mother, she was happy with my correct answers. She said, "Everything you are saying is on the way to Dao." She was teaching me what we did and what we said have to follow the Dao. With Dao in mind, we could achieve it eventually. Sometimes she was saying to me, "You are trying to be fancy again." This was her encouragement for me to make full use of Qi for dealing with different health conditions which I did. I developed quite a few healing methods of my own style that helped many people for their health problems.

'My mother is a kind-hearted person, but also a strict person. Sometimes she was too strict to be accepted. Some of her students left her as they couldn't pass her 'test'. I once asked mother about this and she said, "I can't be too flexible. I have too many people to organise. People come to me with different purposes, some for good name, and some for money. I have to test them. For a period of time, I felt too difficult to pass her test; I was a bit depressed and reluctant to go on trainings with mother. But when I looked around and thought if I wanted to inherit the lineage for the future generation, I had to bear and pass all her tests. Let alone many students had high expectations for me and they relied on me to be the next lineage holder; they gave me a lot of support and encouragement. After ten years learning from mother, particularly with the incomparable relationship as mother and son, the born with connection for sensitive message exchange, I inherited all what mother taught me; the whole serial of Da Yan Wild Goose Qigong system.

'After mother granted the 28th generation lineage holder to me in 1998, she said to me, "Don't be afraid that some people would make trouble. Don't bother some people deny the lineage holder. It is always good to have high level masters in our society. Those who keep the Wild Goose only for themselves will possess nothing. Truth is truth. You can achieve high only when you have high moral standards. You must carry on the teaching task to pass the skills to future generations."

'Da Yan Wild Goose Qigong is the treasure of China, based on the Chinese philosophy, the Chinese culture, the Chinese medicine and has the three in one form. As the 28th generation lineage holder, with moral standard in mind to benefit the society, I travelled to different parts of China for teaching classes, giving lectures in the spirit of promotion for the traditional Chinese culture. This is the best way to inherit the legacy of mother. I will unite all the people who have the common goal with us. I will lead the thousands of students of Da Yan Wild Goose as the backbone of our team, to carry on this cultural heritage of Kunlun Da Yan Wild Goose Qigong for the health benefit of people, for the flourishing cultural developments in China. I think this is the best way for recollection of mother; this is the best way to requite her kindness.'

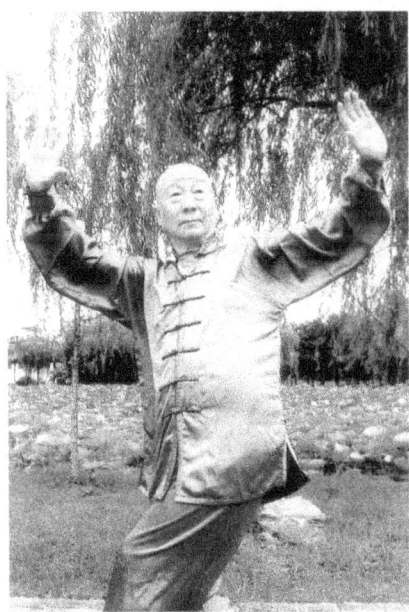 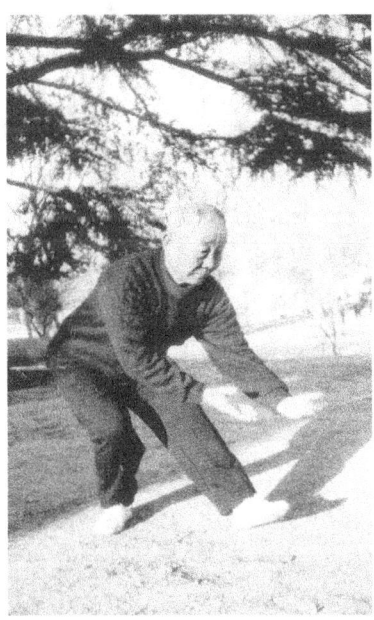

Grand Master Chen Chuan Gang, 28th generation linge holder

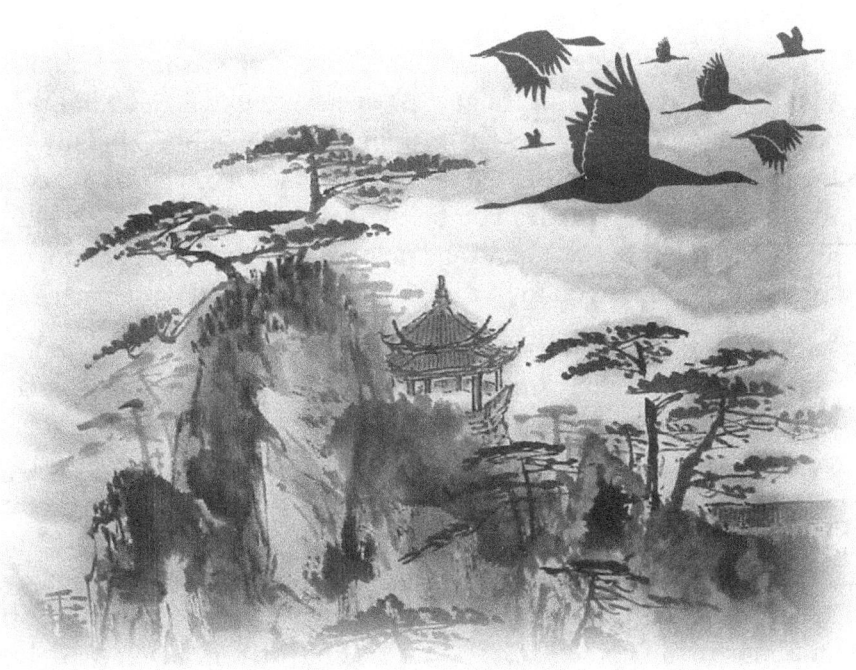

Chapter 4

A Continuing Journey
Into the Chinese Healing Arts

Da Yan - Wild Goose Qigong
The 1st 64 movements

A Continuing Journey into the Chinese Healing Arts

When I started my journey with the Chinese healing arts in 1987, initially it was to improve my health and to gain physical strength and flexibility after a serious accident in 1979. What has kept my interest and become my passion was the underlying principle and philosophy of the Dao. The Dao encourages you to live life fully; it guides you on the path to an enjoyable, healthy and fulfilling life. Nothing is beyond it and no one can avoid it. It does not remove you from life; it guides you to live well at all times in all circumstances.

I have been working on myself for thirty-five years. In the first four years, this work was more on the external or physical level with orthopaedic doctors and physiotherapists. I found them to be friendly and professional, but they offered no long-term suggestions or solutions. I remember very clearly when the Professor of Orthopaedic Surgery I had seen for three years told me that I would have to plan for early retirement at the age of forty, as the injuries that I had sustained would lead to severe arthritis to most of my body. His parting words when I left his office for the last time in 1983 were: 'If you have too much pain come back and see us and we will be able to give you some medication for it.'

I was not suffering too much pain, just a little bit of cramping and aching in my legs. I was mainly frustrated with my inability to do many physical activities in order to lead what I thought was a normal, active life. As I had suffered fractures to both feet, both ankles and both legs I could not be involved in any running sports or a lot of other activities. I remember going to parties and nightclubs dancing with my friends in my early twenties; it was always a lot of fun. But I would have to pay the price the next day. It would feel like I had two badly sprained ankles and could hardly walk for most of the day. I became very careful about doing too many physical things and knew there had to be a better way.

I wanted to discover more of the internal aspects of my life. I had spent fifteen weeks in hospital when I had the car accident in 1979, although I have little memory of the first three or four weeks. But what I experienced was a sense of peace; a complete feeling of nothingness and this is what I wanted to realise more of. Once I started meditation practice in 1984, my internal world became alive and my true identity started to emerge. Through regular meditation and other psychotherapy practices, I have been able to identify and let go of suppressed emotions and other energetic blockages which were limiting my growth. One of the main ones: 'Why me, why did this have to happen to me?' is a common question and an emotion that people feel when they are recovering from an accident or serious illness.

I feel very fortunate or maybe it's just destiny that I have been given the opportunity to do the work that I do. Without the hardships and obstacles that have come my way, I wouldn't have learned the skills required to first heal myself, then to help others.

When I started my journey into the Chinese healing arts in 1987, I felt an immediate affinity with this ancient healing practice. The gentle movements and energy releasing exercises had an instant effect on my stiff joints and tight muscles. As I continued my study and research into the Chinese healing exercises, it became clear to me that this was a way of increasing and maintaining my mobility. Since 1992 when I became a full-time teacher, I have been practising some type of dynamic (movement) or static (meditation) practice three to five times per day, five to six days per week. My strength and flexibly has increased and I don't have pain in the joints or other problems in this area.

From about 2004, I had pain in my right foot; a nerve was pinching between the metatarsal joints whenever I was standing or walking. After consulting a number of natural therapists over a few years, it was diagnosed as Morton's Neuroma and was caused by my badly broken right femur (thigh bone) which was turning my right leg in and creating excess pressure on the foot. The only long-term solution was to have surgery and cut out the nerve. I hadn't seen any orthopaedic doctors since 1983 and my local doctor encouraged me to have a full examination with a leading foot and ankle specialist in Sydney, Australia. In 2011, thirty-two years after I had the accident, I was armed with a complete set of new X-rays of all my old injuries. The doctor and I discussed my medical history and how I had been managing my condition. He viewed the X-rays and gave me a full physical examination; his comment was: 'Extraordinary, you have no arthritis.'

It was very clear on the X-rays that there was no inflammation around the joints in my feet, ankles, legs and hip area. According to Traditional Chinese Medicine (TCM), arthritis is a stagnation of blood and Qi around the joints and this would have shown on the X-rays. There was a slight bone on bone in my right ankle and I have been aware of pain and stiffness in this area for many years. The doctor asked me what I did to manage it. I replied that I would do a simple stretching exercise for the Achilles tendon a few times each day to stimulate blood and Qi into the ankle and foot area to relieve the stagnation and thus the pain.

In 2011 I had the surgery to remove the damaged nerve in my right foot and this has been a real relief as it has greatly increased my comfort and mobility. I gave the doctor a copy of my first book *The Art of Life* and explained how the warm up exercises and all the different types of Chinese healing exercises would benefit most arthritic conditions. As I write this book it's been thirty-five years since I had the serious car accident. I'm very pleased that I have had confirmation that the Chinese health exercises that I have been doing, which have become my life over the last twenty-eight years, have been working.

Four thousand years ago in the central areas of China people were practising Qi guiding exercises to relieve the effects of dampness within the body. This area of China around the Yangtze River is renowned as being very hot and humid; these gentle exercises would help clear stagnation around the joints and allow individuals to manage the pain and discomfort of what we call arthritis.

Another important part of the traditional Chinese health program that I have been doing regularly, is the drinking of green tea. Since the mid-1990s I have been drinking one to two pots of good quality green-leaf tea each morning. There have been many studies conducted which indicate that green tea helps relieve arthritis-related inflammation and cartilage breakdown. There have also been many positive studies conducted in recent times about the effects of Chinese exercises (Qigong/Tai Chi) on arthritis and other health conditions. Meditation and other mindfulness practices have also reported favourable outcomes in many scientific studies. Modern research is starting to prove what ancient people have known for thousands of years; how diet, exercise and the state of our mind has a major effect on our health and the quality of our lives.

There are many different types of Chinese exercise or what we call 'Qigong'; which translates to 'working with or cultivating the Qi or life-force energy'. When I commenced my training in 1987, I was mainly studying and teaching martial styles. Firstly a westernised style of Taijiquan (Tai Chi); it had a lot of benefits for relaxation and general health but it was modified and stylised to suit the mainly older population. I wanted to learn the so-called 'real thing' and in 1996 became a lineage student to a traditional Chinese master. I studied Yang style Taijiquan with many martial arts and self defence applications, as well as basic TCM theory, massage and other traditional healing techniques. It was an amazing growth period for me. From 1998 I started to travel to China regularly, (this year 2014, will be my thirtieth trip) leading study groups and attending international Qigong conferences. I was now being exposed to all the different traditional styles of Qigong and I became interested in the history, philosophy and healing benefits of the Chinese medical and Daoist styles of Qigong. By 2002 I had stopped practising and teaching Taijiquan, one of the martial Qigong styles, to focus on studying, sharing and promoting Chinese medical and Daoist styles of the Chinese healing arts.

Meeting the Master

On the 2007 China Qigong study tour we spent a week in Wuhan in Hubei province, central China. We were studying Daoism with Grand Master Cheng Zhen, the Abbot of the Chang Chun or Eternal Spring Monastery. One of the group, Ken Morgan, an acupuncturist from London who was also an experienced Qigong practitioner, had a contact phone number given to him by one of his teachers for the Grand Master of the Wild Goose Qigong who lived in Wuhan. My business partner Jing contacted the master and arranged a meeting with our group. The meeting was arranged at the hotel we were staying at; the master arrived with his wife and he appeared to be a gentle man in his eighties wearing normal clothes. Before he started talking to us he took off his jacket, then his shirt and trousers to reveal a beautiful pale yellow silk traditional outfit. As he started to talk, which was translated by Jing, you could see and feel the energy glowing out from within him. We were all mesmerised; even the hotel staff who were preparing the restaurant for lunch sat down to experience his amazing presence. He talked about the history of Wild Goose Qigong and how Qigong had grown and developed in China from ancient times. He answered all our questions and gave an inspiring demonstration. They could not stay with us for lunch as they had another engagement, so when they were leaving I gave him a small gift and also one of my Qigong DVDs. He gave me one of his DVDs and with a beautiful smile said, 'You all always welcome to come to Wuhan and study Da Yan Wild Goose Qigong with me.'

In my travels to China I had met many great masters at international conferences, at TCM universities and hospitals, and visiting Daoist and Buddhist masters at the sacred mountains. They had all enhanced and helped developed my own understanding of Qi energy. It does take a long time to refine your own energy; traditionally it's called practising 'Gong Fu' (Kung Fu) which translates to 'the time it takes to cultivate or master a skill'. It can take many years of practice as well as working out ways to incorporate it into your life. The ideal is that it becomes natural, not just something you are quoting from books or what your teacher has said. Through the work, our own energy is refined and through the laws of attraction the right people seem to appear to help us on our continuing journey. I was not interested in learning more styles of Qigong; I was coming to the end of a huge project of publishing three books as companions to the three DVDs that I had already produced. I was very happy and content with the Qi cultivation methods that I working with and my life had become very busy leading many workshops and retreats on these practices.

Having met Grand Master Chen Chaun Gang, the 28th generation lineage holder of the Da Yan Wild Goose Qigong, I realised it was not my decision. It was destiny that we had met and everything since then has fallen into place. The Da Yan Wild Goose Qigong is a proud historical treasure of Chinese culture and I feel very honoured that I have had the opportunity to study with the 28th generation lineage holder. I don't think I would have been ready either physically or mature enough twenty years ago or even ten years ago, to understand and fully comprehend this ancient healing system.

I was aware of this style of Qigong and had read a few articles about its history. I had the opportunity to learn a modified Wild Goose Qigong form in the early 1990s and it didn't feel right then, but it felt right now. In 2009 I returned to Wuhan with a group of twenty enthusiastic students. We had beginning students as well as Qigong instructors from most areas of Australia as well as the United States and the United Kingdom. For seven days Master and Madam Chen with a group of six of their senior students expertly taught us the 1st 64 movement set. It can be difficult learning with a large group as everyone can have a different interpretation. This can lead to misunderstandings about the correct form and this is how some of the Chinese exercises have changed when they have gone to other countries.

I returned to Wuhan in 2010 for two weeks' private training with Master and Madam Chen. I had been in Beijing attending a Qigong conference and travelled down to Wuhan afterwards. It was early July and it was very hot and humid; Wuhan is renowned as one of the furnaces of China. The morning sessions were outside and in the afternoons we would go to their apartment which had air conditioning and we would move the furniture and continue training. One of their students Vivien who had very good English would translate. I would practise with one of the senior students with the master watching every detail. We had breakfast, lunch and dinner together and they wanted to know everything about me; my Qigong training history, my family history going back a few generations and what my plans were for the future. I meet their son, daughter and son-in-law and many of their students; they made me feel very comfortable as if I was being welcomed into their extended family.

We spent the first few days revising the 1st 64 movement set that was taught to me the year earlier. I had been practising regularly and teaching it to one of my groups in Sydney. I felt very confident with the movements, but they made a lot of adjustments to my form. It wasn't until 2012 when I had been back another two times that they were happy that my form was 100% accurate. As I mentioned earlier, this can be a problem learning in a large group. I was very pleased to then learn the 2nd 64 movement set directly from Master Chen in all its fine detail. Master Chen has an amazing energy for a man of his age, but I was concerned that he should not do too much or get too tired and waste his Qi. I discussed my plans to bring smaller groups to study with him. I would lead and instruct the group and he would give the finer details and add more insight. We organised advanced training groups in 2011, 2012 and 2013 with future groups being planned.

The Da Yan Wild Goose Qigong is an amazing set of exercises; it has been researched and developed for over a thousand years, then handed down from one generation with respect and purpose to the next. It improves our health and quality of life on the physical level, as well as on the emotional level, giving us the opportunity to connect on a spiritual level with the divine. Once our energy comes back into balance or our Qi is in order, we return to our natural state which allows us to fully experience the beauty of the world we live in. I feel very fortunate that I have been given this job or opportunity to help others on their healing journey; the teacher or educator is held in high regard within traditional cultures. I look forward to learning more and sharing all that I know so others can benefit.

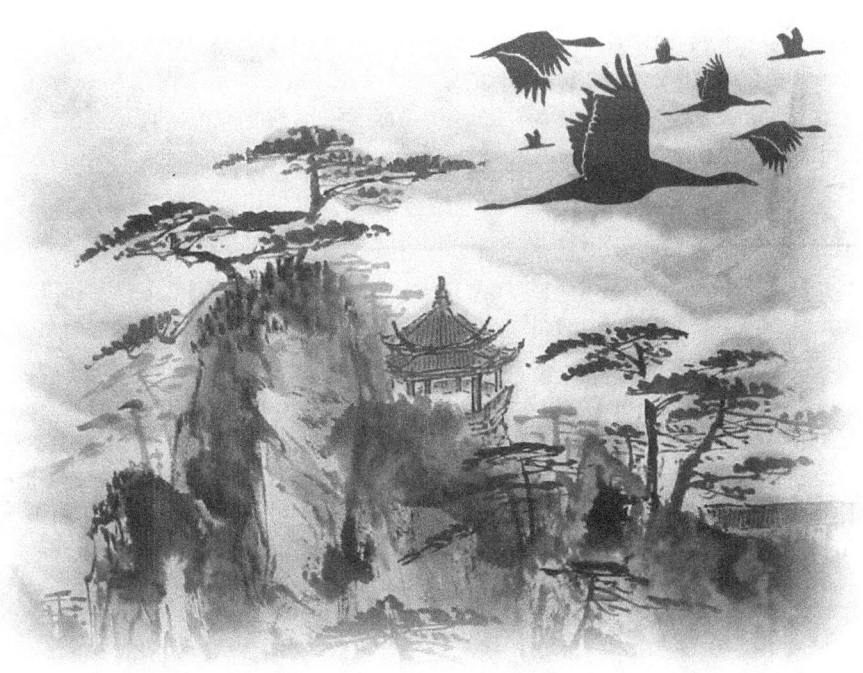

Chapter 5

The Art of Practice

Da Yan - Wild Goose Qigong
The 1st 64 movements

The Art of Practice

To get the most out of your practice there are a few basic principles and guidelines as well as precautions that you should be aware of. These principles are important for gaining a deeper understanding and realising the full benefits of this ancient healing art. Proper practice ensures positive results and eliminates potential negative effects.

Relaxation and tranquillity are the fundamental requirements and methods for Qigong practice. From the external to the internal, we first start by relaxing the physical body as this helps relieve respiratory and mental tension. Tranquillity means allowing the mind to be calm and find inner peace; the practice of tranquillity in Qigong requires quiet external surroundings and a peaceful internal world. Internal tranquillity, with your mind relaxed and focused, is more important than external silence. Relaxing can induce tranquillity while tranquillity helps relaxing. Complete relaxation is possible only when complete tranquillity is present.

Correct practice helps induce the effect of relaxation and tranquillity, whereas incorrect postures may inhibit one's ability to realise this state of relaxation and tranquillity. Correct postures and movements take time to master and are dependent on the individual's specific physiological and psychological characteristics at their stage of practice. The difficulty and intensity of practice should be adjusted according to the person, the time, the place and their attained state, in order to produce the desired mental and physical relaxation. Otherwise, improper practice may produce only stress and fatigue.

Making it a pleasurable experience as you progress from beginner to advanced level, is a fundamental principle in learning Qigong. We should practice persistently over a long period of time; Qigong practice is a process of constant accumulation. As long as one perseveres with the practice, the effects will be obtained gradually and naturally. Some students show significant improvements within a short period of time, whereas some practitioners do not display any distinctive changes for a long time, and some may start with positive effects which soon diminish. Whatever the effects, it is important to have a correct and positive attitude. Being confident about oneself and persistent in practice are important. Qigong is a practical method, and long-term practice is the only way to get real effects. It's common to experience different sensations when practising Qigong. Feeling warmth and a tingling sensation in different parts of the body is common, as well as the rising of emotions and some people even report seeing different colours and visions. Try not to have too much attention on sensations as it can deplete your Qi experience. It's better to go to the level of no sensation to return to nothingness.

The Philosophy of the Wild Goose
The wild goose is a high energy bird which flies thousands of kilometres from one side of the world to the other and over 10 000 meters high up over the mountains. It is very graceful, as well as being proud and honourable. It's also very protective of its flock. When we practise we try to adopt some of these characteristics, as this will increase our Qi field and make practice more enjoyable.

In ancient Chinese and Egyptian cultures the wild goose was considered a messenger between heaven and earth. In India the wild goose is known as the 'vahana' or the vehicle for which Brahma the Hindu God of creation travels on. It's also associated with the sun, prana (Qi), knowledge, atman, spirit and the creation of life itself. In China, geese are still a symbol of marriage and long life; in rural communities a newly married couple would be given a pair of geese as a wedding present to signify their bond of marriage. In the Roman Empire, the wild goose was the sacred animal of Juno, the protector of women and the goddess of light, marriage and childbirth.

The Ganalbingu or the Magpie Goose people, the ancient indigenous inhabitants of central Arnhem Land Australia, have lived in harmony with their land and environment for thousands of years. The goose, their eggs and their nests are sacred to the Ganalbingu people. Special ceremonies depicting the goose are held for aiding the health of newborn babies and their mothers.

The goose, with its powerful flight and migratory habits, can be associated with travelling. The journey may be difficult, but the goose can help people find perseverance. In earlier times, shamans were aided by spirit geese on their journeys to other worlds. In modern psychotherapy geese are associated with communication or the ability to express oneself. In ancient mythology as in modern psychotherapy, geese are still regarded as symbols of marriage and the importance of a solid, happy home and family life.

During the 1st 64 movement set the goose is resting in between journeys; its feeding and gathering energy preparing for its next flight. In the opening movements we have an image of these birds being happy and having fun. The purpose of these movements is to gather good Qi from all directions and to disperse bad Qi. To become one with the universe. The goose is flying over water (lakes and rivers) and it is feeling happy. It looks for good Qi from the distance, for pure Qi; grasping it for increased energy and preparing for its next journey. Playing with the Qi ball brings good Qi into the body. Then the goose descends as it looks for water and food. It continues to process and refine Qi after its all-day activity, then it finds its way back to the nest before dark and goes to sleep. During the 2nd 64 movement set the goose awakens in the morning and calls on the rest of the flock to embark on a great flying journey. It still exercises during the flight to regain energy; it gathers good Qi through its eyes from looking at the sun, moon and Milky Way.

The Five Aspects of Naturalness
When practising, Grand Master Chen advises that we follow the five requirements of naturalness:

1. **The naturalness of mind.** 'Exercise with no guidance from the mind. Have a free and empty mind without deliberately clearing it, because it can always be clear as long as no attention is paid to it.'

2. **The naturalness of breath.** 'There is no need to regulate the breath. Just follow its natural flow. The breath will be regulated after the aura or Qi field is open and clear.'

3. **The naturalness of body.** 'Keep the knees straight in a natural and relaxed way. Relax the face and let down the shoulders and elbows. Relax the waist and hip and keep the chest slightly open without folding it or humping the back. Clear the Ren channel and lift the back to let the Du channel run smoothly.'

4. **The naturalness of metabolism.** 'With the mechanism of exercises, the stale Qi inside can be exhaled from the body and the primordial Qi, or Yuan Qi can be inhaled so that the acupoints and the channels can be cleared and the aura or Qi field can also be motivated. As a result, the internal organs can be nourished, which will speed up the process of the merging of the natural Qi and the primordial Qi in the body.'

5. **The naturalness of exercise.** 'Keep a relaxed and quiet state of mind. There is no need to pretend, as the right state of mind will come during the exercise. Place the tip of the tongue on the roof of the mouth to link the Ren and the Du channel and let the body fluid flow back down to the diaphragm. Keep the eyes steady with the light outside and the spirit inside. As a result, there will come the state of emptiness and the Qi outside will naturally be inhaled. And at this moment the mind will follow the movement, which is the so-called unity of movement and mind. All the movements from the start to the end of the exercise make up the cycle of motivation, circulation, enhancing and gathering of the vital Qi inside the body, which will bring a great balance and an overall effect to the function of the body. The naturalness of exercise also means that the Da Yan Qigong is suitable for people of all ages.'

The health and healing benefits

There are many health and healing benefits associated with regular practice of the Da Yan Wild Goose Qigong. Within the instruction sections of the 1st and 2nd 64 movement books, both the anatomical and energetic benefits for each movement are listed. Theoretically each individual movement will benefit a specific area or condition, but it is the accumulation of practising the complete set of exercises from the beginning to the end many times, when the real benefits will be realised. From my own experience and the feedback that I have received from my students, the many bending, twisting and stretching movements aid in blood circulation, flexibility and balance as well as overall strengthening of the whole body. Please read the inspiring stories sections in both books, telling of individual's own experiences of practising these Chinese healing arts for many years.

Meditation, processing the Qi

Our thinking mind uses the most energy of our body; when the mind is calm and relaxed it can increase our energy, whereas when the mind is very active it can deplete our energy. After practising the dynamic moving sections of the Da Yan Wild Goose Qigong, we practise the static or stillness section. This part of our practice is very important; when the body comes to a complete stop, the Qi keeps moving and through the tranquillity of the mind, the Qi will come into order. It's what we call the 'processing' stage; it's important to keep your thinking mind out of the way and to allow the Qi to do its work. The movements clear the meridian system, dispelling stale Qi and absorbing good Qi, helping foster Yang with tranquillity breeding Yin. To balance Yin and Yang we need a good balance between dynamic and static; too much movement or stillness by itself can unbalance Yin and Yang.

Where and when to practise

The wild goose always flies the same route so it can find its way home again. So try to do your practice at the same time and at the same place. The goose is fussy and choosey when coming back to the nest. It likes to make it cosy for a good night's sleep, ready for the next day's journey. Practising in one regular location will create and form a Qi field and this will improve your Qi development. I remember one time we were practising with Grand Master Chen before breakfast and it was raining and we couldn't go outside to our regular spot. We found a spot under cover near the hotel and Master Chen led us in Goose Walking; we walked around in a circle with our arms away from our body similar to the commencing movement for a few minutes. This created a Qi field on our new practice area; once we had cleansed the space we began to practise.

It's important when we start our practice to face towards the western direction if this is possible; this is because the structure of the movements are based on the Five Elements. The different directions relate to the elements and their corresponding meridians and organ groups of the body. The Da Yan Wild Goose set moves in all directions while absorbing the Qi from the Five Elements and the universe. This accumulative effect builds the Qi in the body. There are many stepping and walking types of movements used for balancing Yin and Yang; each time the foot presses the earth it is Yin and each time it releases it is Yang.

When we start as new students, it's important to practise with a group, as the flock works together to help each other. This group energy also creates a strong Qi field that everyone benefits from. Another way is to attend regular retreats and intensive training sessions, which also increases your Qi field. In time we can practise on our own to master the movements and make them our own.

Exercising in the early morning and late afternoon when the sun rises and sets is a very powerful time, as there is a natural transition between the dark coolness of night (Yin) and the bright warmth of day (Yang). The setting of the sun and transition between Yang and Yin is also a time when nature has a great influence on your body. You might notice that birds are very active at this time of day, as they are in the morning. It's important not to look directly into the sun in the early morning or late afternoon, as this can cause damage to your eyes.

Qigong can be practised anywhere, but some places are better than others. You should be undisturbed during Qigong practice to help maintain concentration in the mind. The best places are in nature in the open air where the heaven (Yang) and earth (Yin) Qi are most abundant. Practise in the mountains or beside a waterfall or the ocean; near water is excellent because moving water generates a lot of Qi.

If you are practising indoors, try to find a quiet and peaceful space away from draughts with natural light and fresh air. Avoid excessive noise, TV sets and computers and turn off your mobile phone or set it to silent.

The proximity of some plants should also be avoided. The Oleander plant for example, is known to be poisonous and has a very tense Qi. As you practice you will learn which plants feel relaxing and harmonious. Lovely flowers and large old trees are ideal.

As a rule, you should not exercise on a full or empty stomach. Instead of eating breakfast, consume liquids as they stimulate stomach-intestine movement which acts as an internal massage. Warm or room temperature water is the best with a slice of lemon, but not cold water from the fridge, as this interferes with Qi circulation.

Qigong exercise in the evenings is a way of freeing your mind and body from the burdens of a busy day; a way of processing the events of the day and letting things go, physically and emotionally. Students often comment on how they get their best night's sleep after attending class. You are able to sleep more quietly and recover more fully because the body begins its recovery during Qigong and this continues during sleep.

We are all a bit different, so I wouldn't advise anyone practising just before going to sleep as it stimulates your energy and may disrupt your sleep. But a few students have told me that when they haven't been able to sleep, they would get up and practise Qigong to calm their mind and body, then have a restful sleep afterwards.

Eating and drinking

For Qigong exercise you need a clear head. Beverages such as alcohol, tea and coffee affect concentration and your body's functions. If you are not calm and relaxed you will not feel the full benefits from Qigong exercise. It's best to avoid drinking cold fluids during or immediately after practice as this interferes with Qi circulation.

You should not exercise on either an empty stomach or after a full meal. Being distracted by hunger will not help your mental focus, so if you are hungry have something light to eat or something to drink. A full stomach interferes with Qi circulation. The Qi is diverted into the digestive system as stomach juices increase and stomach-intestinal movements occur, leaving very little Qi to circulate elsewhere.

When not to exercise

When we exercise we absorb the good influences from nature and the macrocosm. Similarly, we assimilate the influences from turbulent weather conditions. Therefore, it is not good to practise Qigong during bad weather, heavy fog, extreme heat, before or during a thunderstorm, on excessively windy days, or during lunar or solar eclipses. Exercise can begin again when nature is balanced.

Menstruation and pregnancy

Qigong is good to practice during menstruation and pregnancy as it will improve the circulation of Qi, blood and other bodily fluids.

Women who are menstruating should pay attention to the effects of Qigong exercise. If the exercise produces a negative effect, stop immediately and continue at a later time.

Special care is also required during pregnancy. Each woman's pregnancy is different and it is recommended that the expectant mother consult her primary care provider as well as a qualified and experienced Qigong teacher.

What to wear

There are no rules regarding clothing but since relaxation is important in Qigong, try to wear loose comfortable clothing, ideally made of natural fibres such as cotton or silk.

If you are limited in what you can wear, for example if you are at work, loosen your collar and tie, your belt or waistband and remove uncomfortable or high heeled shoes. It's important that you wear flat soled shoes or even bare feet are OK. I always wear soft sports shoes as I damaged my feet and ankles a long time ago and I find wearing shoes gives me a bit more support. It's a personal preference and there are many light soft shoes available that are suitable.

Whatever clothing you choose to wear, it should not be tight around the waist because the Qi needs to flow easily. Preferably, remove watches and bracelets as they restrict the flow of Qi through the wrist.

If it is chilly, dress appropriately. Feeling cold during a Qigong session can decrease the effectiveness of the exercises, particularly if your hands, stomach or back are cold; chilling your kidneys severely restricts your Qi circulation. I often start my practice on colder mornings with gloves, hat and a warm jacket; you can always take them off when you heat up.

How long to practise

The benefits that are gained from Qigong are proportional to the amount of practice undertaken. The Da Yan Wild Goose Qigong 1st 64 movement set takes approximately ten minutes to complete. It is recommended practising three times through, for a total of thirty minutes at least once a day. It is only when the body's carriage is regulated according to Qigong principles that the Qi will flow easily and the benefits of Qigong realised. If you can achieve thirty minutes twice a day, you will notice a marked increase in vitality and peace within a few weeks. If you have major health issues and can manage a couple of hours per day, you will soon see a radical improvement in your health and wellbeing. Regardless of your state of health when you begin, any amount of regular practice will improve how you feel.

The 2nd 64 movement set of Da Yan Wild Goose Qigong also takes approximately ten minutes to complete. When you are comfortable and have mastered both the 1st and 2nd 64 movement sets, Grand Master Chen advises that we practise the 1st 64 movement set twice, followed by the 2nd 64 movement set once, for a total of thirty minutes twice a day.

How long does the effect of Qigong exercise last?

Qigong works because the Qi is brought into order and the mind, body and spirit are in harmony. This harmony can be disturbed by arguing, getting excited or annoyed, engaging in strenuous physical activity, eating excessively and even going to the toilet. If possible, use the toilet beforehand rather than after Qigong exercise because urination and defecation bring the Qi into definite motion.

I often tell my students after a Qigong class that if they have driven a car there not to play the radio when they leave, as all your senses have been enhanced and the body functions are in harmony. You may get good ideas, solve some problems or if you are with friends you may have amazing conversations. Look at the beauty of the sky, trees and the divine in all living things; I love to look at clouds. It's a creative time, so use it and the Qi will be with you longer. The more you cultivate your Qi the more in harmony with the universe you will be, improving all aspects of your life.

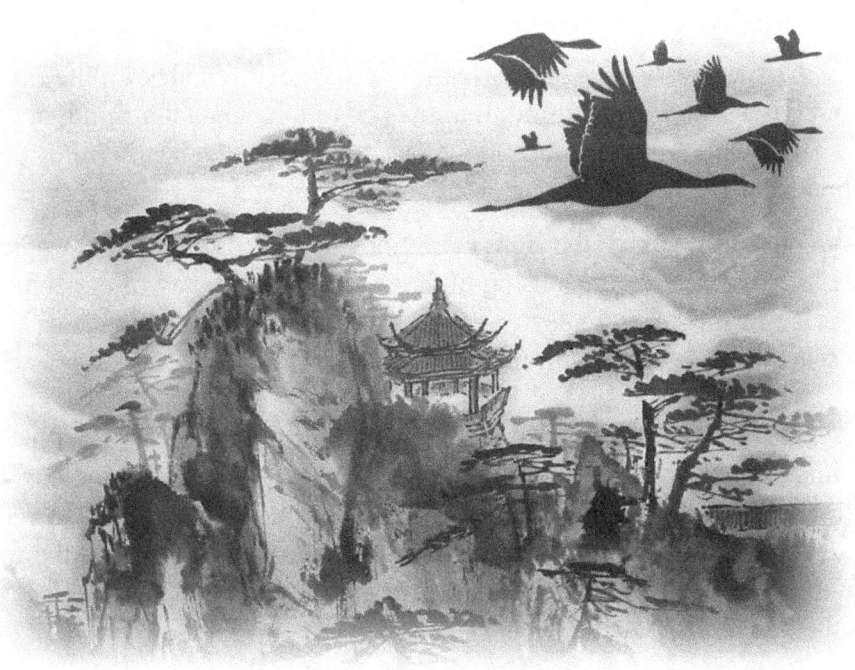

Chapter 6

Qigong Preparation Movements

Da Yan - Wild Goose Qigong

The 1st 64 movements

Qigong Preparation

Qigong is a cultivation exercise which benefits the physical body, the energetic or Qi body as well as the mind. It allows us to rebalance our mind, body and breath and with regular practise it enables us to create a healthy lifestyle and to identify our true spiritual nature.

It is important to create the right conditions before, during and after practice to get the best results. According to the ancient Daoist way of understanding our relationship and connection with the universe, we allow our internal landscape to harmonise with the external landscape.

Da Yan Wild Goose Qigong is a very dynamic set of movements with a lot of bending and stretching. It is important to prepare the mind, body and breath before we start to practice. Qigong practises abide by the basic principles of the three adjustments or three tunings. It is a way of calming the mental activity of the brain and turning on and tuning the mind to tune into the breath and the body.

- **Tuning the Mind**
- **Tuning the Breath**
- **Tuning the Body**

Qigong should never be practised when you are feeling physically cold, energetically cold or emotionally cold. The Qi will not flow very well and can even have an adverse or harmful effect. Good preparation is equally as important as good practice and a good close.

The warm-up is not only a way of preparing the mind and body for the Qigong movements that follow, it is also very good exercise. Physically, when we loosen and rotate the joints, we exercise the ligaments and tendons as well as the membranes which secrete synovial fluid to lubricate the joints. This can improve many arthritic conditions. Energetically, we clear stagnant energy (Qi) that can accumulate around the joints. The stretching movements also help stimulate the meridian system as well as strengthen the muscular system. According to Traditional Chinese Medicine (TCM), the Qi draws the blood through the body. So when we stimulate the Qi circulation we also stimulate blood circulation.

Generally, when we have finished the warm-up, we feel warm, tingling and have turned on and tuned into the body, breath and mind.

Preparing the mind

During the preparation and warm-up we first concentrate on the mind and allow the excess Yang energy or activity of the brain to descend down. When we have too much activity in this area it can be very hard to concentrate. We keep our mind in the present moment by initially concentrating on the flow of the breath. In time the breath will become smooth and even and this will allow your mind to rest.

When we are in this relaxed state we can use our intention and direct our awareness, like the light of a torch, on each part of the body as we are exercising it, from head to toe. Through this active meditation we consciously awaken the body by feeling and seeing what we are doing.

Preparing the posture and breath

Keep the body upright with the head and spine naturally in alignment; allow the muscles and flesh to relax around the skeleton. The movements of Qigong help clear the energy blockages in our body. With time and practice the movements will become natural and effortless.

There are a number of different breathing patterns for different styles of Qigong. For the styles presented here, we will breathe in and out through the nose to the abdominal area, slowly, deeply and naturally. When we breathe in, the abdomen gently expands and when breathing out, it gently contracts. This is known as natural breathing. In time, the breath will naturally coordinate with the movements, helping the mind to focus and allowing a fusion between mind, body and breath.

Basic stance

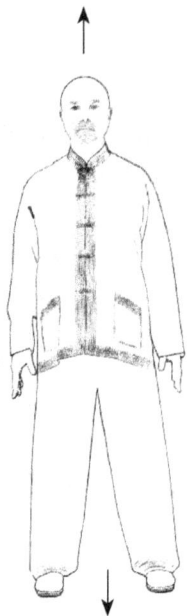

Stand with feet parallel, shoulder-width apart, as if standing on train tracks, with the knees slightly off lock. Let your weight sink into your legs, feet and into the ground. Keep the coccyx or tail bone slightly tucked in, chest relaxed, and the back straight. Hold your arms away from the body. Fingers are open and relaxed and pointing to the earth; palms are facing the body.

With the chin slightly tucked in and the top of the head (Bai Hui point) reaching to the sky as if a silken cord attached to it is lifting the whole body, lift the Hui Yin, gently squeezing the pelvic floor. Relax your eyes and face and look out into the distance. Keeping your jaw relaxed, place the tip of your tongue on the top palate of your mouth, just behind the front teeth. Breathe in and out through the nose. When breathing in, let the abdomen push out slightly and as the breath goes out, let the abdomen come in. Just relax, letting the whole body breathe.

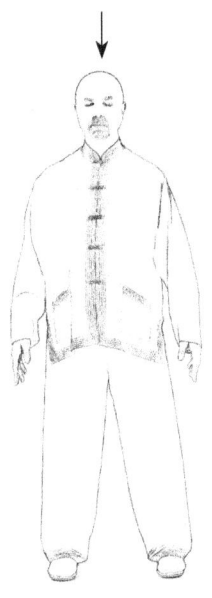

With the eyes closed, allow the breath to become smooth and even, and let your mind rest. After a few breaths, concentrate on the out-breath, relaxing from the top of the head to the soles of the feet. Just relax down through the body on the out-breath. After a few more breaths, let the knees and hips sink a bit closer to the ground, feel the pressure go into the feet. Like a tree, follow the roots from the soles of your feet deeply into the ground. As you let the breath out, relax down through the body into the ground, letting the stress and tension of the body dissolve into the earth.

After another few breaths, with your awareness, push up the spine one vertebra at a time, checking that the chin tucks in a bit and letting the head pull away from the body. We seem to stand taller as the top of the head reaches up and touches the sky. Stay in this posture for a few breaths, feeling the peace. With your eyes gradually opening, look out into the distance, but not looking.

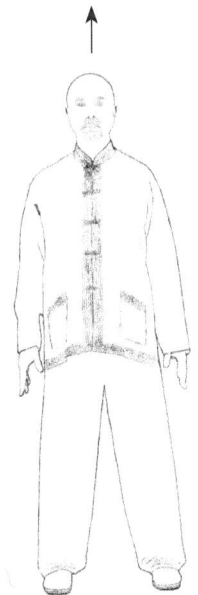

The Warm-Up Movements

Arm and chest stretch

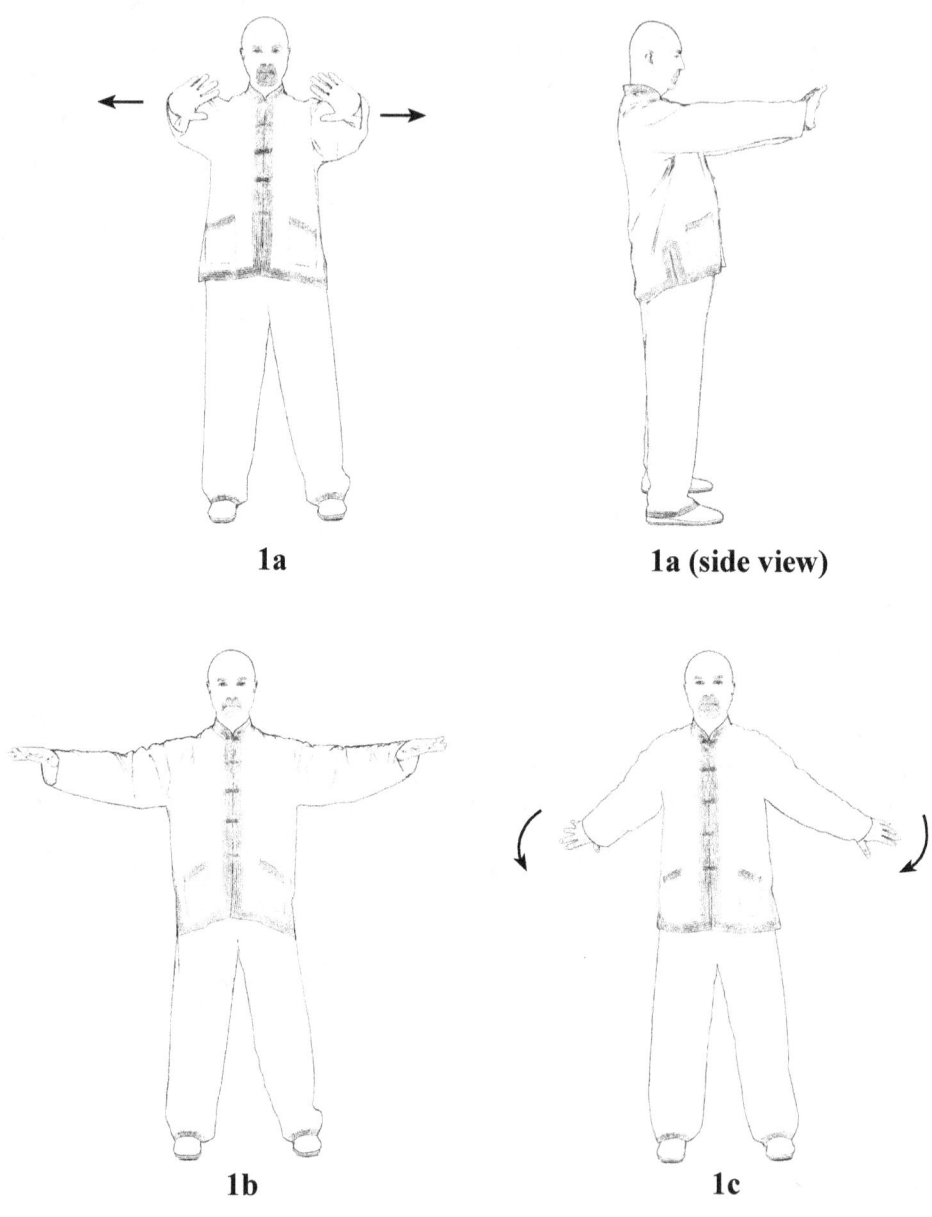

1a-c Raise both arms up in front of the body to about shoulder height. Turn your palms out and push to the sides, feeling your chest and rib cage open. Push back and stretch back as far as comfortable.

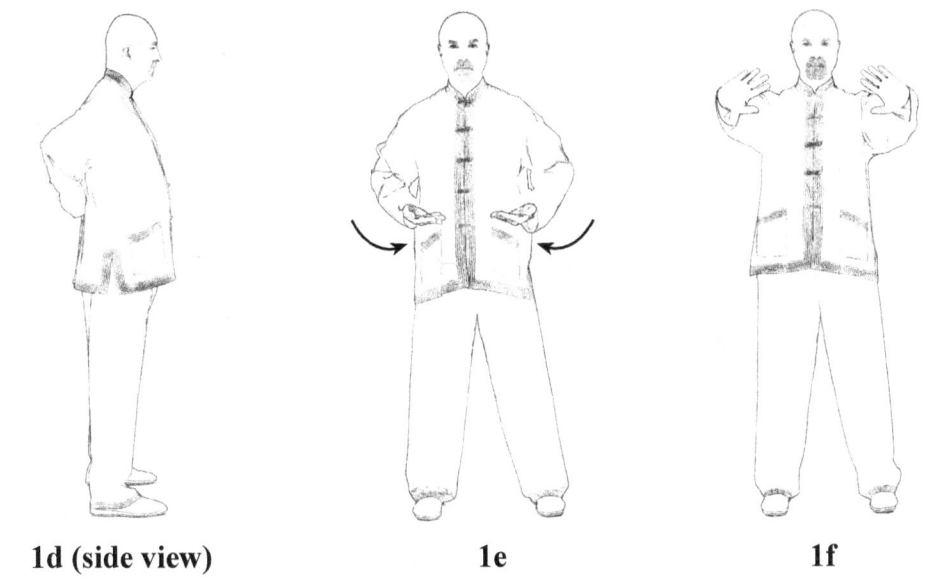

1d (side view)   **1e**   **1f**

1d-f   Turn your palms up, bend the elbows and bring hands to the front of body brushing by the waist. Repeat 4 times, similar to swimming breaststroke.

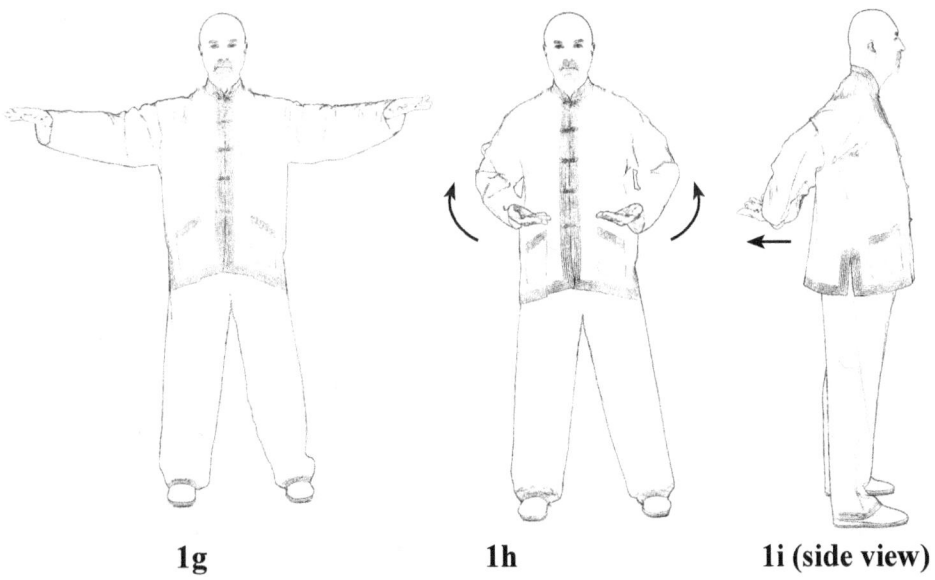

1g   **1h**   **1i (side view)**

1g-i   Then repeat four times in the opposite direction: with palms up, hands brush by your waist and stretch behind; slowly rotate palms and bring arms in front of the body.

This movement exercises the chest, shoulders, elbows and wrists.

Body roll

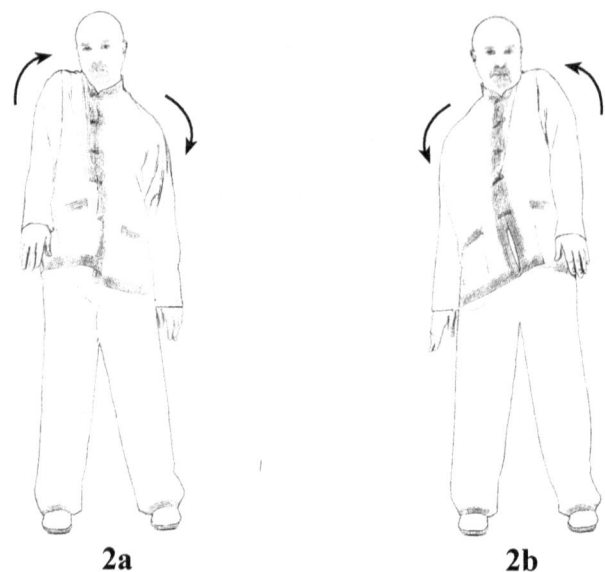

2a **2b**

2a-b Let your arms slowly descend to your sides. Slowly roll one shoulder and then the other, like swimming backstroke. With your awareness, feel the motion massage your shoulders, chest, your abdomen, and your back over the kidney area.

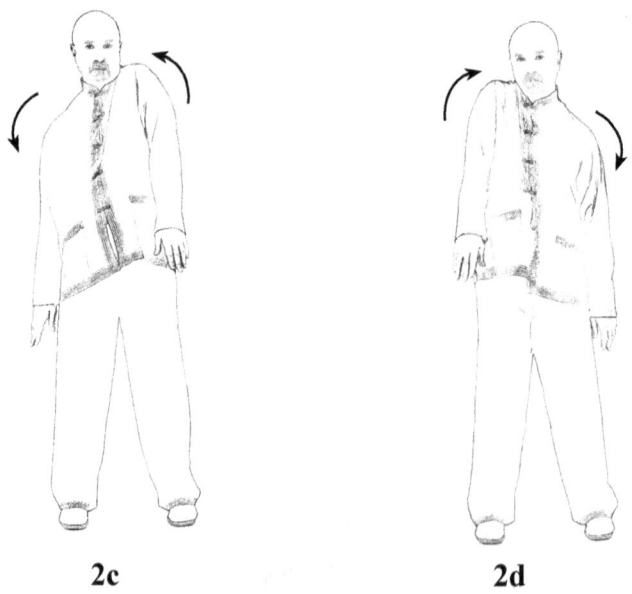

2c **2d**

2c-d After about 8 rotations, stop and come back the other way, rotating forward, and feel the internal massage.

Hip rotations

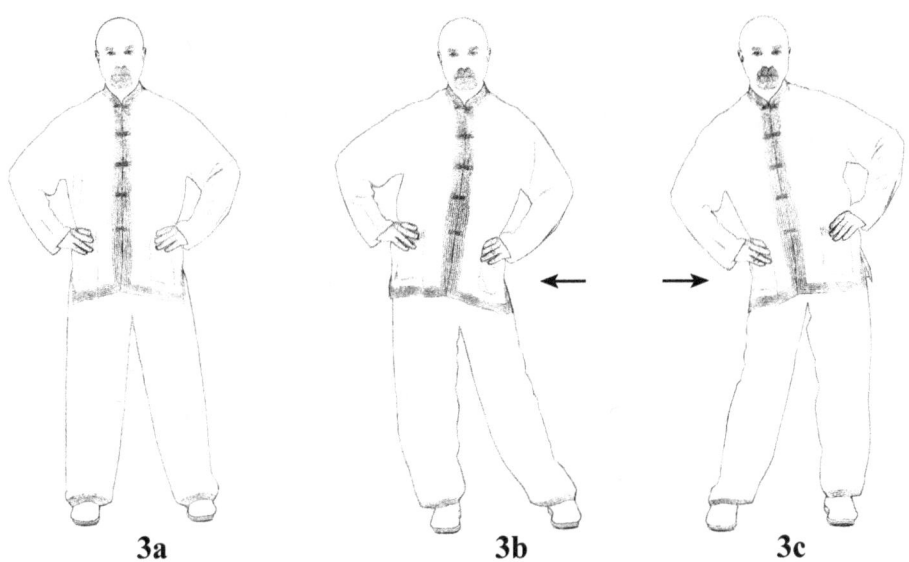

3a **3b** **3c**

3a-c   Place your hands on your waist and start to move your hips from side-to-side. Relax and feel the movement of the hips.

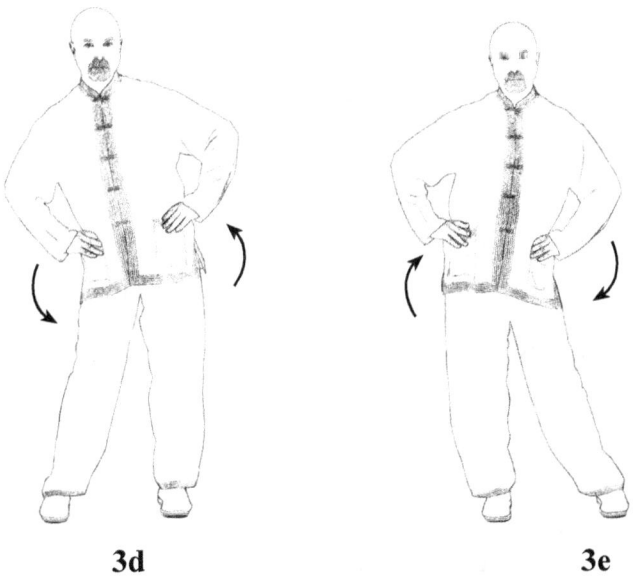

3d **3e**

3d-e   After about three movements to each side, start to move the hips in a circle, gradually increasing your range of movement. Follow the spiralling movement up the spine to the top of your head. Feel and see the movement of the hips. After about 6 rotations, stop and come back the other way.

Walking and massaging the feet

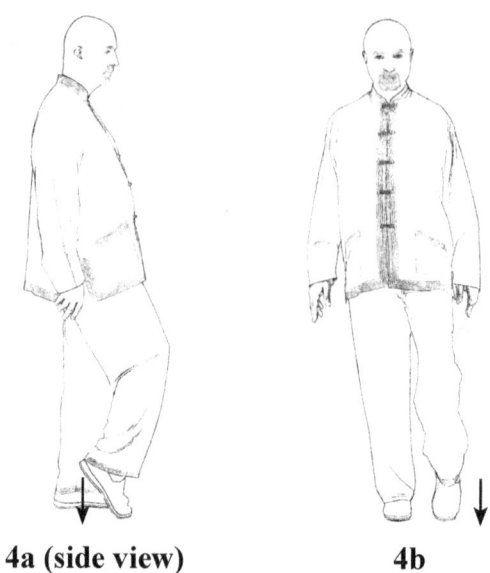

4a (side view)   **4b**

4a-b   Stand with your feet closer together, walking on the spot. Push firmly from the toe to the heel six times to each side, letting the weight of the body massage the feet. Feel and see the tendons, muscles and joints of the feet.

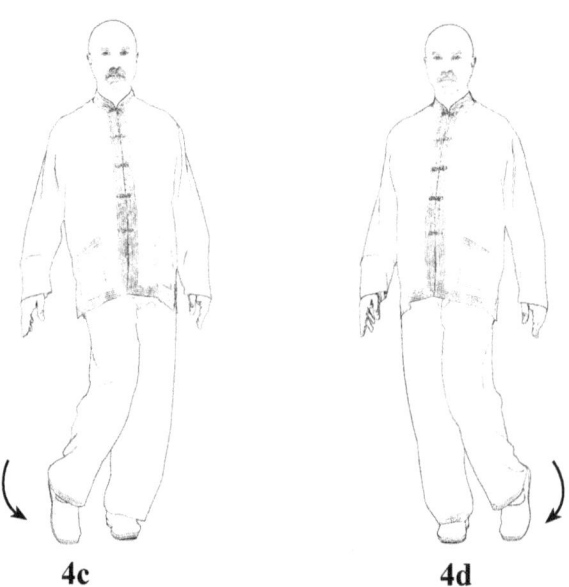

4c   **4d**

4c-d   Turn and twist while moving your knee across the body, massaging the inside of the foot on the floor towards the big toe. Repeat about six times to each side.

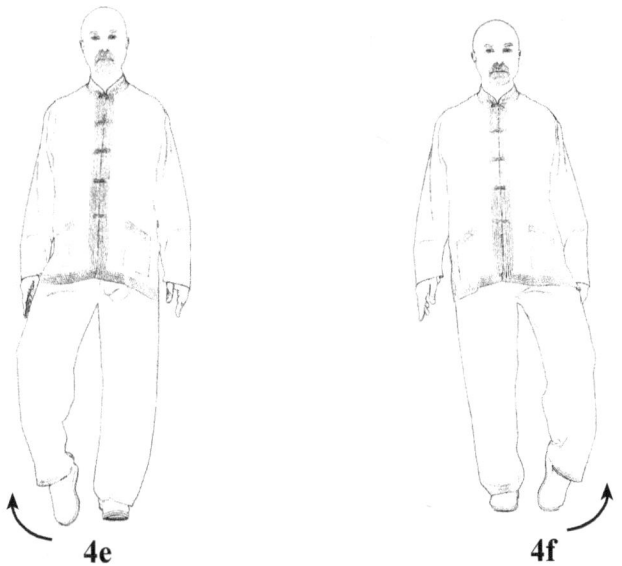

4e   **4f**

4e-f   Stop and push to the outside of the foot, massaging towards the small toe, 6 to each side. Relax, feel and see the movement of the foot.

Shaking the legs

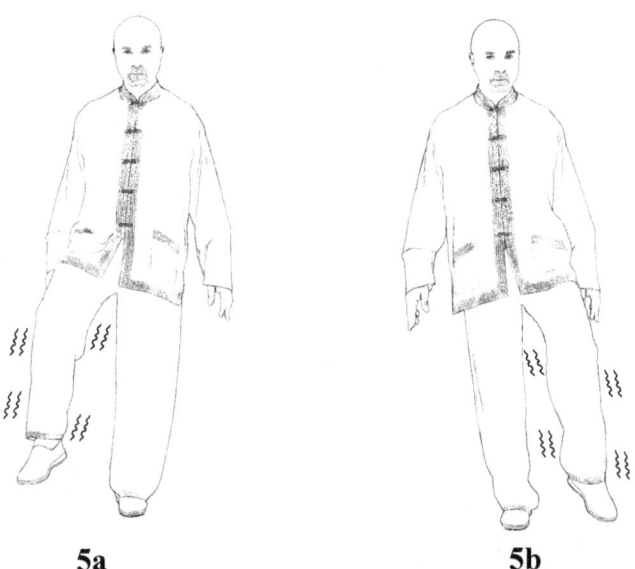

5a   **5b**

5a-b   Shake your legs three times to each side, allowing the Qi and blood to flow.

Hand and wrist shaking

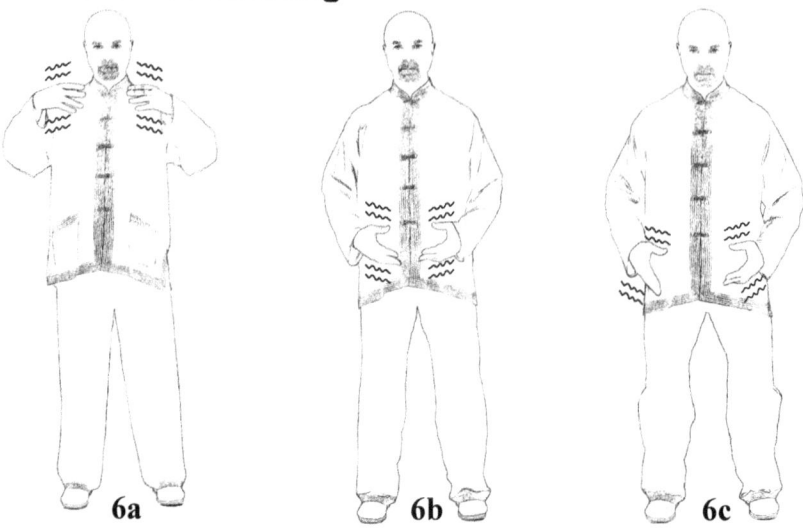

6a-c   Shake your hands, up and down about 6 times, loosening the hands.

Back and front stretch

With any type of stretching movement always start gently and then gradually increase your range of movement. With time and practice you will be amazed at how your flexibility will increase.

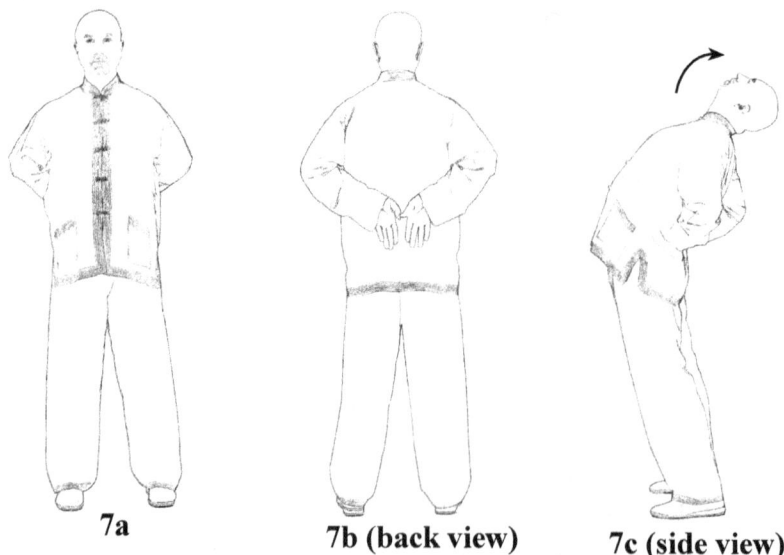

7a

7b (back view)   7c (side view)

7a-c   With your feet parallel, and about shoulder-width apart, place the back of both palms onto your lower back. With your legs straight, gently lean back; only go as far as feels comfortable. With your palms supporting your back, pull your elbows back and gently stretch across your chest and shoulders. Your eyes are looking up towards the sky. With each out-breathe stretch a little more. Continue for a total of four breaths.

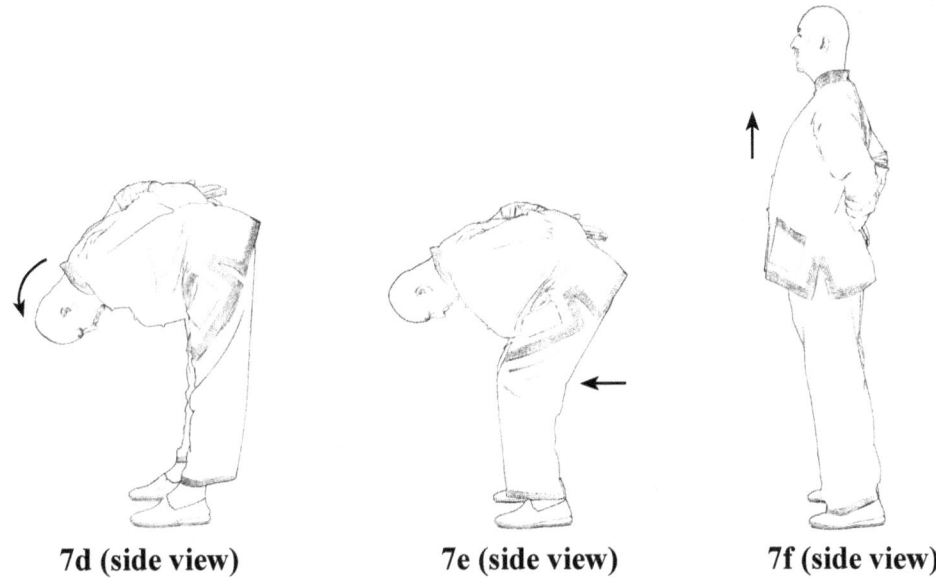

7d (side view)   **7e (side view)**   **7f (side view)**

7d-f   Push your hips back and swing your body forward. Keeping your legs straight and bending from the waist, lean forward and gently fold the body in half. Only go as far as feels comfortable. The eyes are looking between the legs. Gently bend your knees and slowly straighten your back lifting your upper body from the waist. Keeping your shoulders and neck relaxed, with your chin on your chest and eyes looking at the ground. It is important to raise the neck and head last after, the body is upright.

Repeat back and front stretch a total of four times.

Side stretch

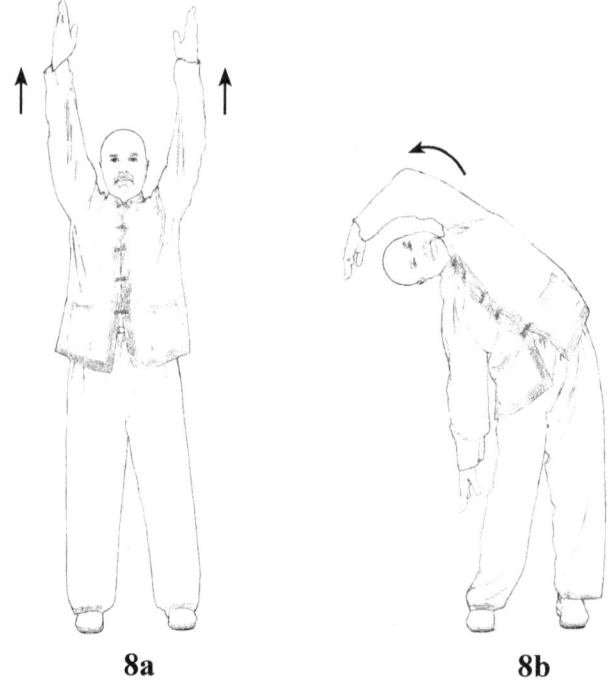

8a   **8b**

8a   With feet parallel and about shoulder-width apart, raise both arms up above your head. The palms are facing each other and the fingers are pointing to the sky. Stretch up, lifting your spine.

8b   Lower your left arm to the side of your body and lean to your left with your right arm circling over your head; fingers are pointing towards the ground and your eyes are looking towards the sky. With each out breath stretch a little bit more. Continue for a total of four breaths.

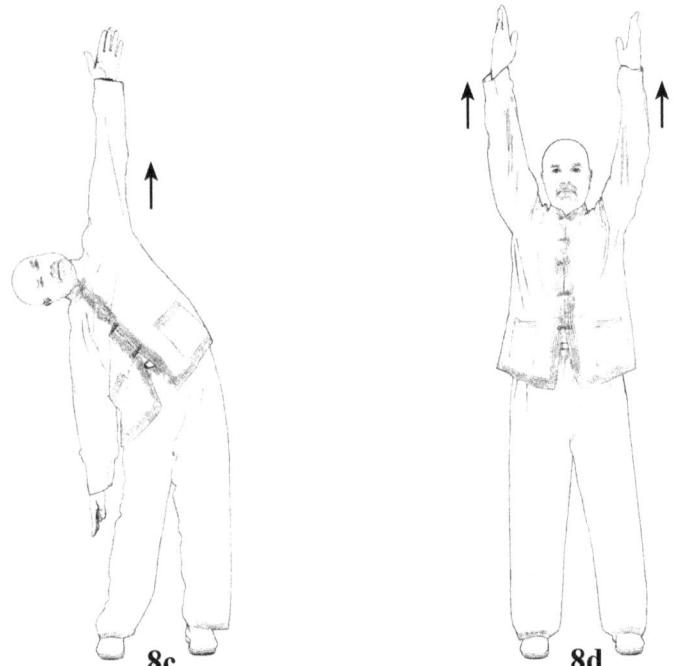

8c-d   Raise your right arm up over your head and then raise your left arm. With the palms of your hands facing each other and fingers pointing to the sky stretch up, lifting your spine.

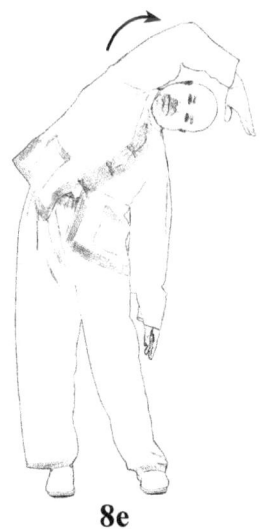

8e   Lower your right arm to the side of your body and lean to your right with your left arm circling over your head; fingers are pointing towards the ground and your eyes are looking towards the sky. With each out breath stretch a little more. Continue for a total of four breaths.

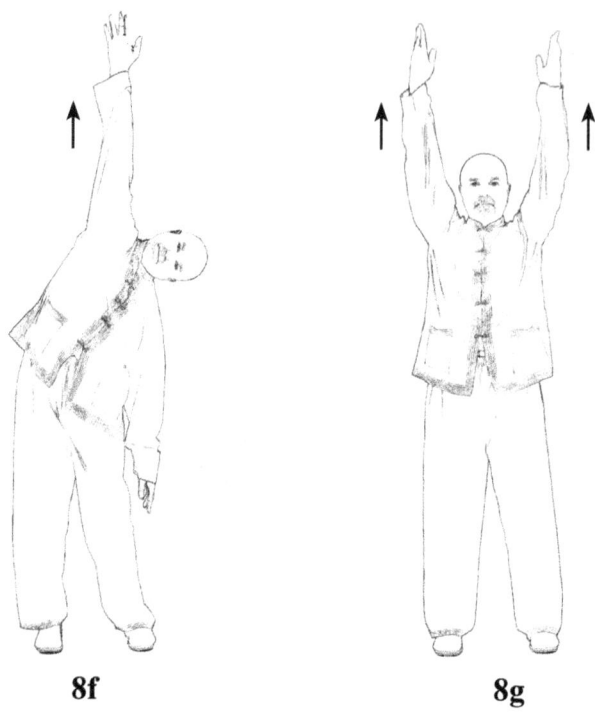

8f   **8g**

8f-g   Raise your left arm up over your head and then raise your right arm. With the palms of your hands facing each other and fingers pointing to the sky, stretch up, lifting your spine.

Repeat side stretch four times to each side.

Front stretch

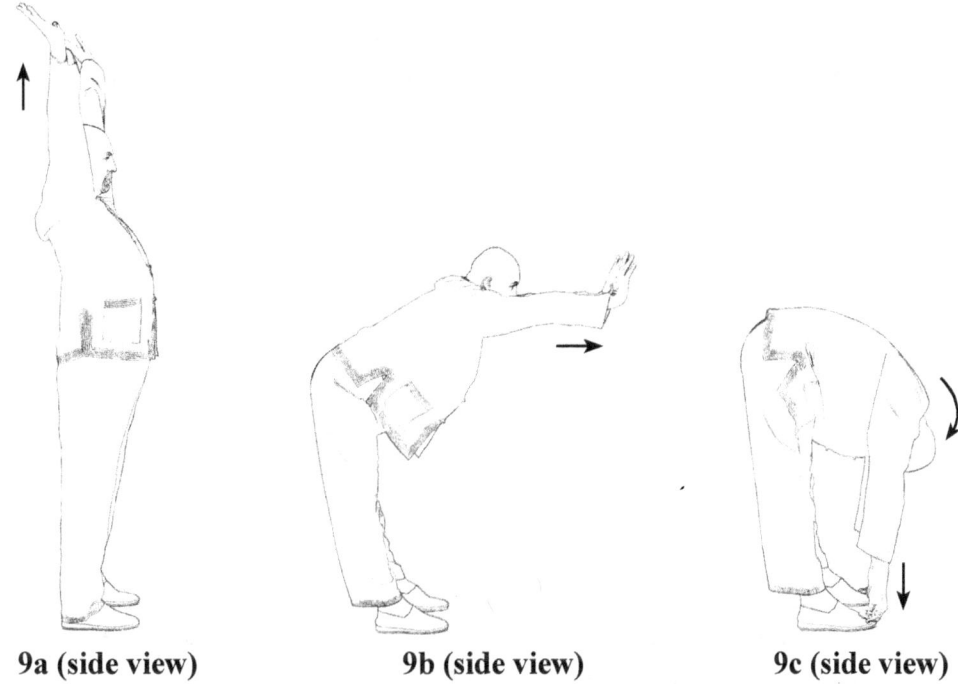

9a (side view)   **9b (side view)**   **9c (side view)**

9a   With your feet parallel and about shoulder-width apart, raise both arms up above your head. Pull the fingers of both hands back, pushing both palms up towards the sky. Stretch up, lifting your spine.

9b   Push your bottom back and lean forward, keeping your legs straight. With your fingers still pulled back, stretch forward, pushing both palms out and stretching your spine.

9c   Bend from your waist and fold in half. Keeping your legs straight allow your arms to naturally hang in front of your body with the knuckles of your hands resting on your feet. With each out breath stretch a little more. Continue for a total of four breaths.

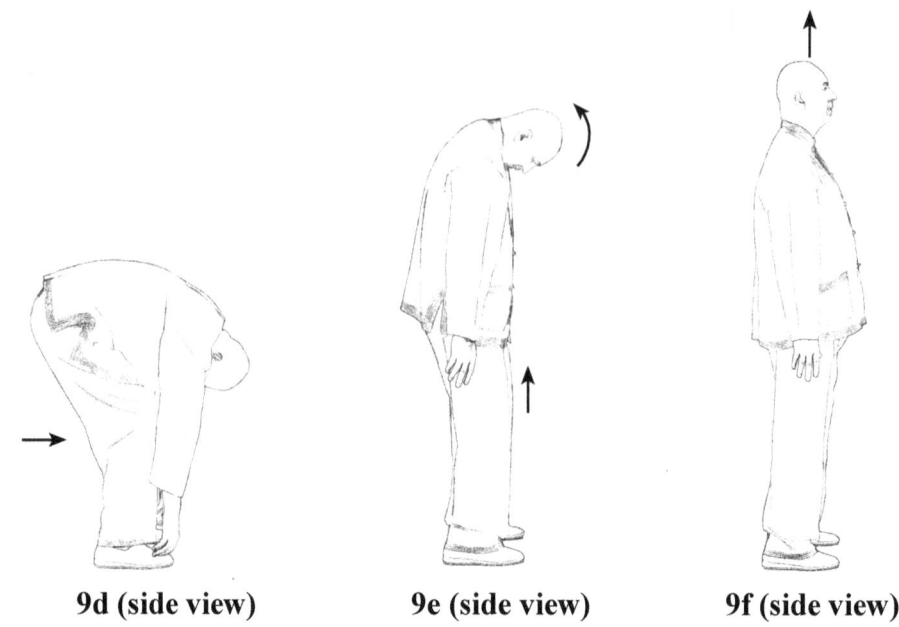

9d (side view)   **9e (side view)**   **9f (side view)**

9d-f   Gently bend your knees and slowly straighten your back, lifting your upper body from the waist. Keep your shoulders and neck relaxed, and the chin on your chest. Your eyes are looking at the ground. It is important to raise the neck and head last, after the body is upright.

Repeat front stretch four times.

Body roll

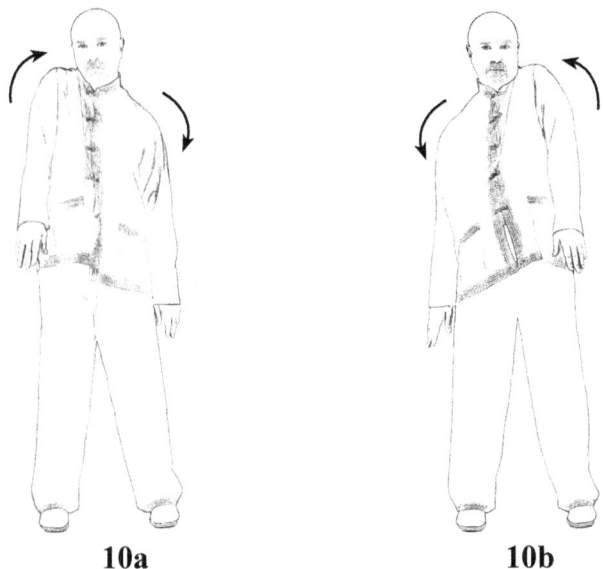

10a   **10b**

10a-b Let your arms slowly descend to your sides. Slowly roll one shoulder and then the other, like swimming backstroke. With your awareness, feel the motion massage your shoulders, chest, your abdomen, and your back over the kidney area.

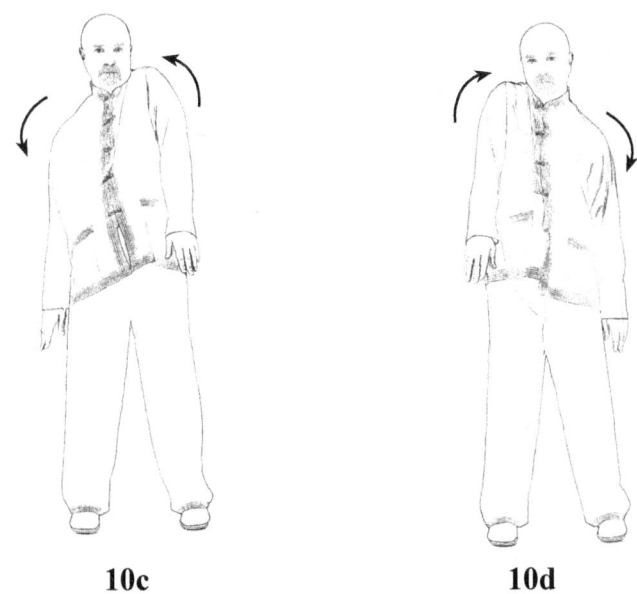

10c   **10d**

10c-d After about 8 rotations, stop and come back the other way, rotating forward, and feel the internal massage.

Body swings

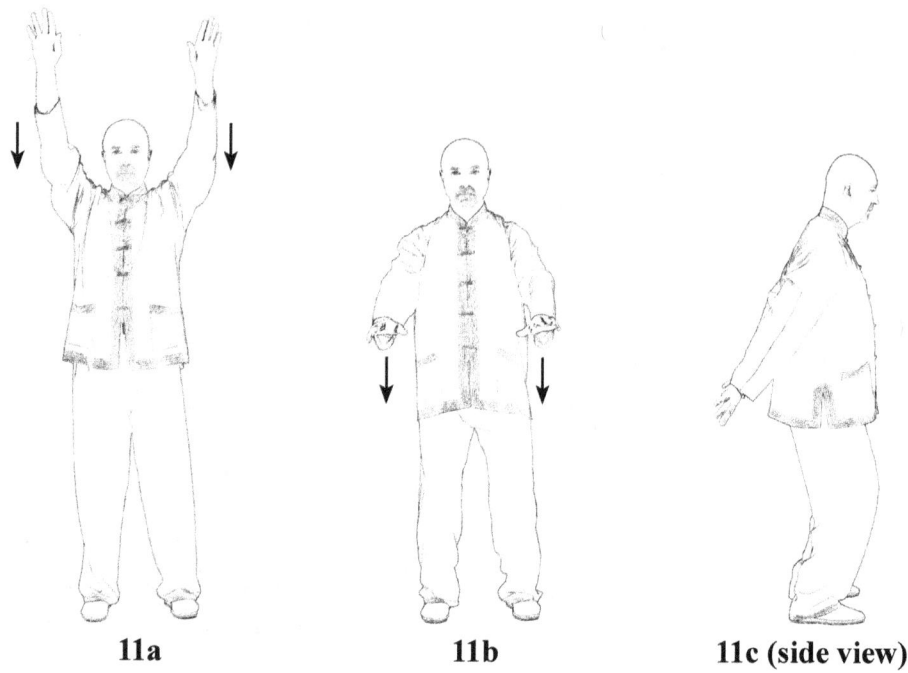

11a   **11b**   **11c (side view)**

11a-c With the feet parallel and arms above the head, swing the arms down, sinking the knees at the same time. Let the whole body swing; keep the back straight and head upright. With your awareness, relax the shoulders and hips, elbows and knees, wrists and ankles, hands and feet. Do this for about 12 swings. This helps strengthen the whole body and is good for blood circulation.

Swinging arms

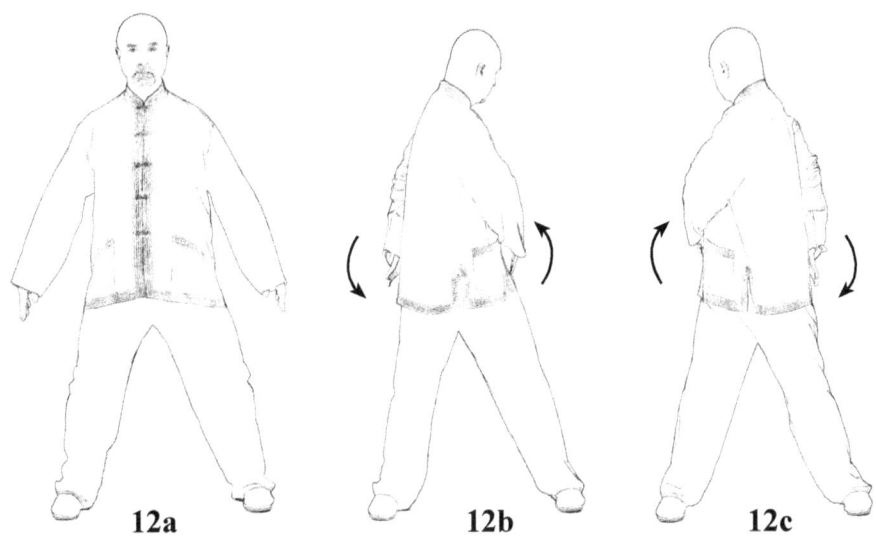

12a-c Step out to a wider horse-riding stance. With the legs grounded firmly and the arms relaxed, let your arms swing out, turning from the waist. Let the arms slap across the body, massaging around the waist and hips.

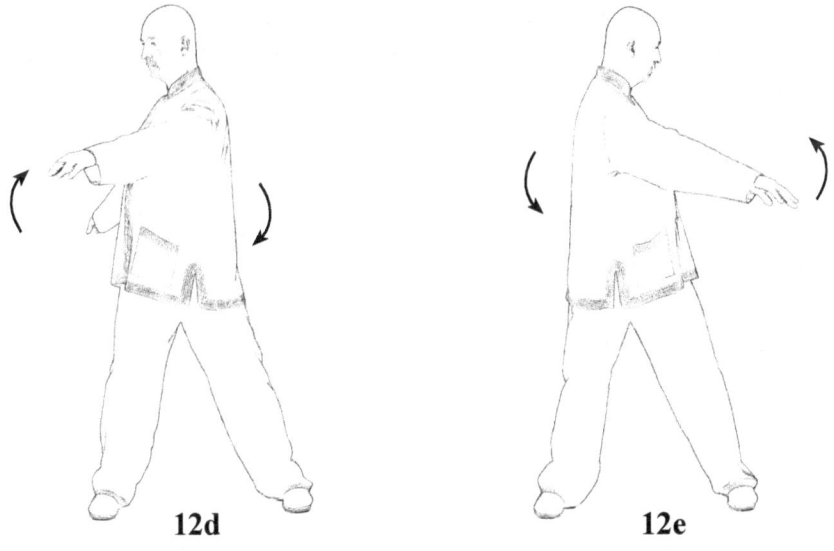

12d-e Let your arms swing higher, massaging around the kidneys and finally, higher again as one swinging arm taps the shoulder while the other taps the kidneys. Do this 12 times.

This helps loosen and strengthen the back and massage the internal organs.

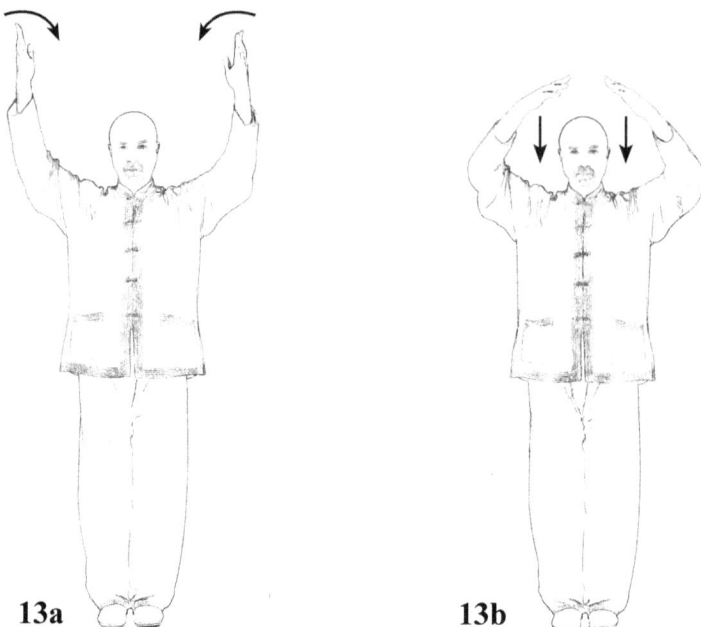

13a **13b**

13a-b Stand with your feet together; raise your hands up above your head guiding the Qi down the body from the top of the head to the soles of your feet. Your arms rest naturally at the side of your body. With your eyes closed, relax from the top of your head down to your hands and down to your feet; relax down through the body on the out breath. Stay in this position and allow the Qi to settle for a few minutes.

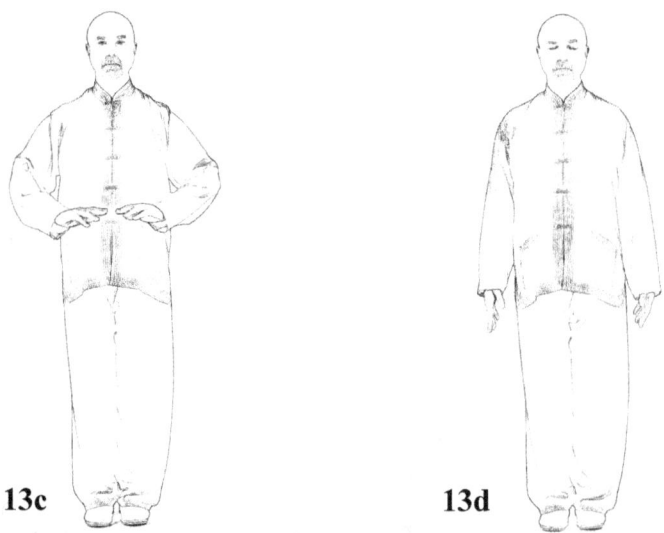

13c **13d**

13c-d With your eyes closed, relax from the top of your head down to your hands and down to your feet; relax down through the body on the out breath. Stay in this position and allow the Qi to settle for a few minutes.

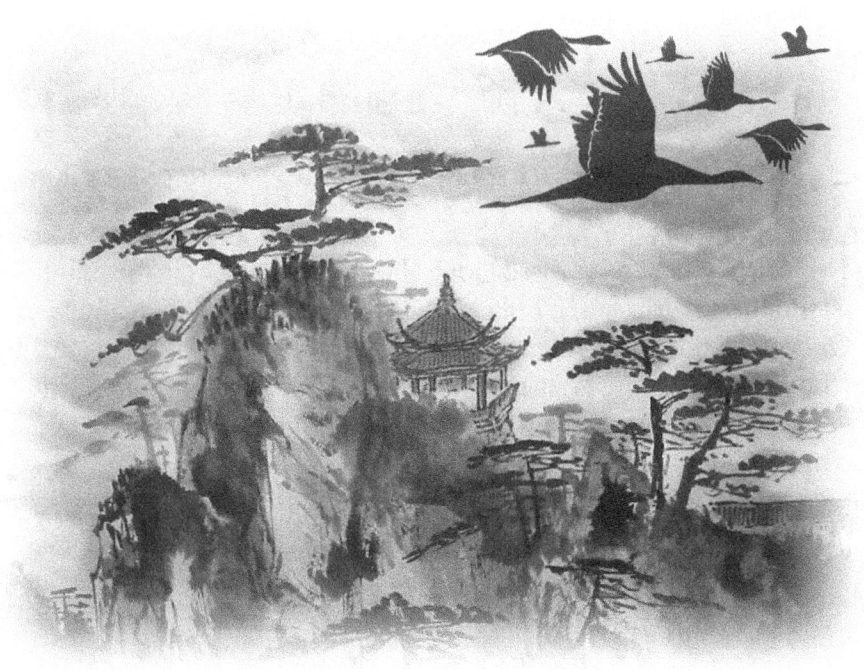

Chapter 7

The 1st 64 Movements

Da Yan - Wild Goose Qigong
The 1st 64 movements

Da Yan – Wild Goose Qigong
The 1st 64 Movements
大雁气功前64式

1. Starting position 起式 Facing the Western direction.

Standing in this position allows the Qi to flow through the whole body, from head to feet. Connecting the Lao Gong (Pericardium PC8) in the middle of the palm with the Huan Tiao (Gallbladder GB30) on the side of the hip stimulates the Qi down the Gall Bladder Channel. Opening the chest stimulates the Qi Hu (Stomach ST13) just beneath the collar bone, allowing the Qi to move down to the Huan Tiao (hip) and down to the Yong Quan (Kidney K1) at the soles of the feet.

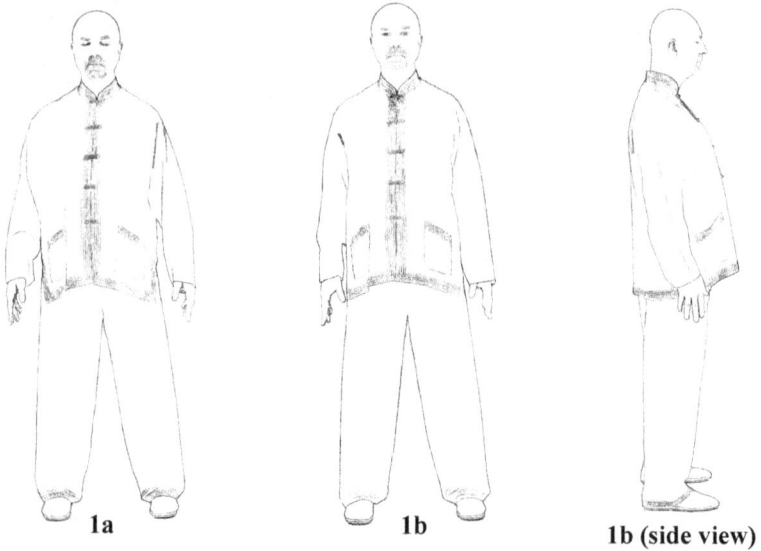

1a   1b   1b (side view)

1a. With your eyes gently closed, stand upright. The jaw is relaxed with the tip of the tongue placed gently on the roof of the mouth, just behind the front teeth. Breathe naturally in and out through the nose. The shoulders are relaxed, arms rounded and palms are facing the body. The hands are relaxed and the fingers are open and slightly curled. The legs are straight with knees slightly off lock and with feet together. With your awareness and breath, relax from the top of your head to the soles of your feet; relax down through the body on the out breath.

1b. Open your eyes and with your awareness focus out to the distance (looking, but not looking). Stay in this position for at least 30 seconds regulating mind, body and breath.

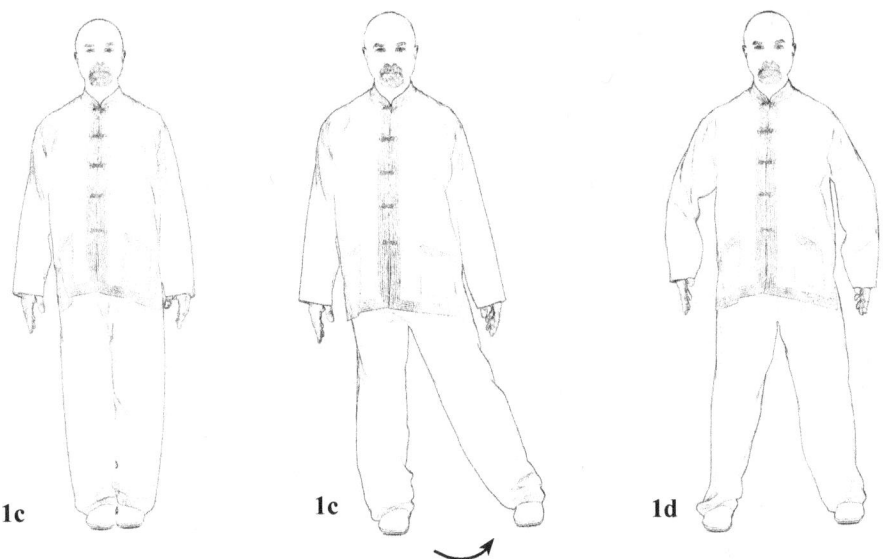

1c   **1c**   **1d**

1c.   Lower the knees and sink down moving your bodyweight slightly to the right. Step to the left by making a small curve on the ground with the left foot. Evenly distribute your weight with your feet no wider than shoulder-width apart.

1d.   Open your chest slightly with your arms rounded away from the body, stimulating the Qi Hu (beneath the collar bone). The Lao Gong (middle of palm) faces towards the Huan Tiao (hip) at the indentation on either side of the buttocks.

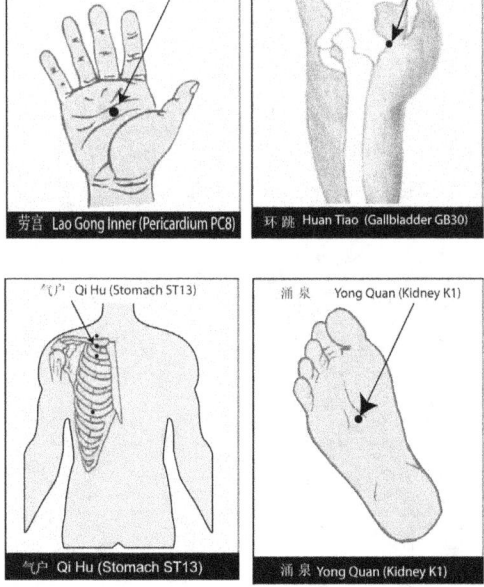

劳宫 Lao Gong Inner (Pericardium PC8)

环跳 Huan Tiao (Gallbladder GB30)

气户 Qi Hu (Stomach ST13)

涌泉 Yong Quan (Kidney K1)

2. Spreading the wings 展翅

When bending forward we are connecting with and gathering the energy of the earth to allow the earth's Yin energy to harmonise with the body's Yang energy. When leaning back we are connecting with and gathering the Yang energy of the sky to harmonise with the body's Yin energy. These movements also open the Kidney and Bladder Channels (Water element) which run up and down the legs and also the Heart and Small Intestine Channels (Fire element) which run up and down the arms. This is important because it is the fusion of the Fire and Water elements, and the connection of Yin and Yang which help to stimulate and open all the energy Channels of the body.

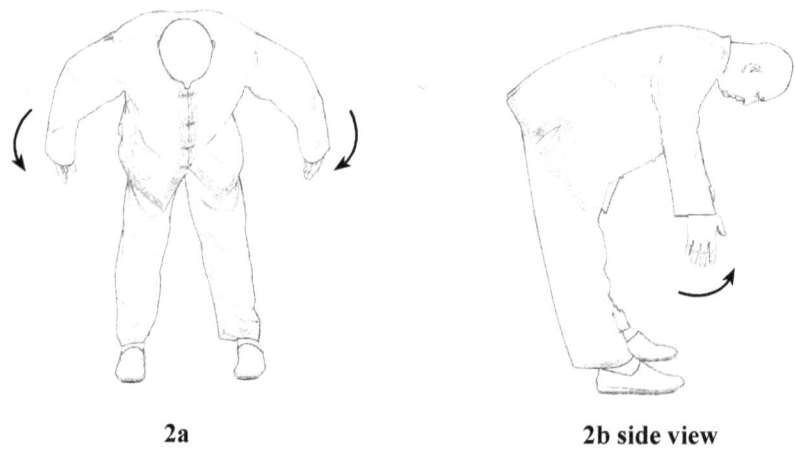

2a   2b side view

2a. From the standing position (1d) move your body forward, bending from the waist 45°. Allow your bodyweight to move onto the balls of your feet, slightly lifting the heels.

2b. Your arms slowly swing forward to knee height as if holding a big ball wider than your feet. The Lao Gong of both hands (middle of palm) face each other. Keep your heels slightly raised, and your weight on the balls of the feet.

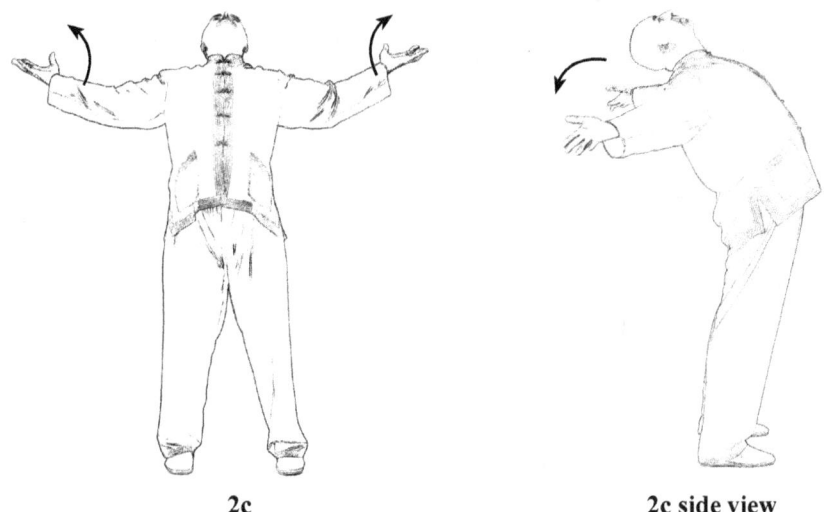

2c   2c side view

2c. Swing your arms back bending from the waist, and as you swing move your bodyweight onto the heels grounding the feet to the earth. Stretch back for two to three seconds and open the chest.

3. Folding the wings 合翅

These movements allow the Qi to gather and accumulate at the Lower Dan Tian (area beneath the navel).

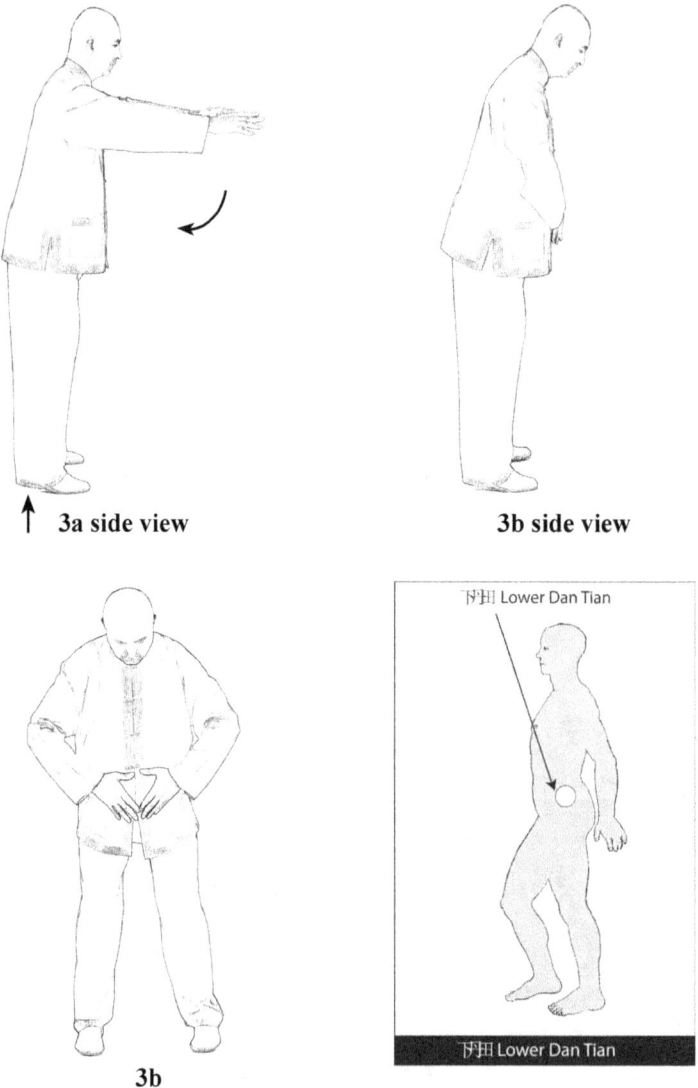

3a side view

3b side view

3b

3a. Swing your arms forward bringing your bodyweight forward and heels off the ground.

3b. With a slight bend at the waist bring your arms to the middle abdominal area. The Lao Gong (middle of palm) faces the Lower Dan Tian (area beneath the navel). The tips of your fingers face each other and the palms are about 3cm to 5cm away from the body. Your eyes are looking forward and down at the earth.

4. Drawing the wings to the back 折窝

Forming the Plum Blossom Claw (four fingers touching together with the thumb) stimulates the meridians which connect five internal organs to particular fingers. We gather this energy at the Kidneys by touching the He Gu (Large Intestine LI4), the webbed area between the index finger and thumb with the Shen Shu (Bladder BL23) behind the navel, either side of the spine beneath the Kidneys. This also stimulates the Bladder and Large Intestine Channels.

Plum Blossom Claw: The five fingers represent the five petals of the plum blossom and when all the fingers are joined, the five elements are united and together they stimulate the five major organs – Heart, Spleen, Lungs, Kidneys and Liver. This is used in many traditional practices within the martial arts and healing Qigong to direct the Qi to a specific area

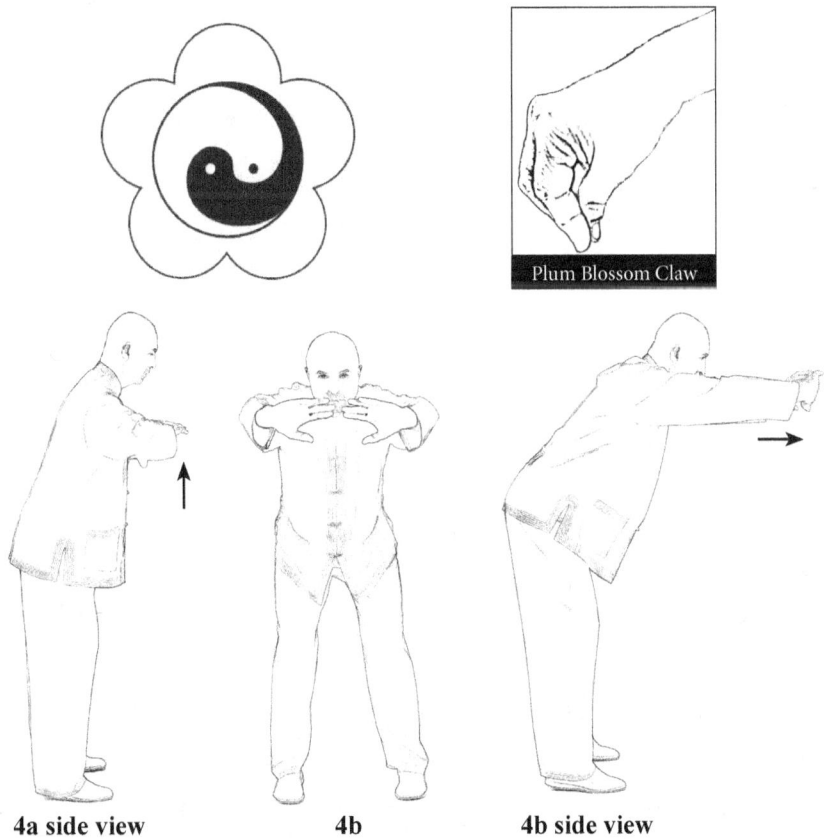

Plum Blossom Claw

| 4a side view | 4b | 4b side view |

4a Gently straighten your back, lowering the heels to the ground. Your eyes are looking straight ahead. With a slight bend at the waist, slowly scoop the hands up in front of your body, with the fingers pointing towards each other.

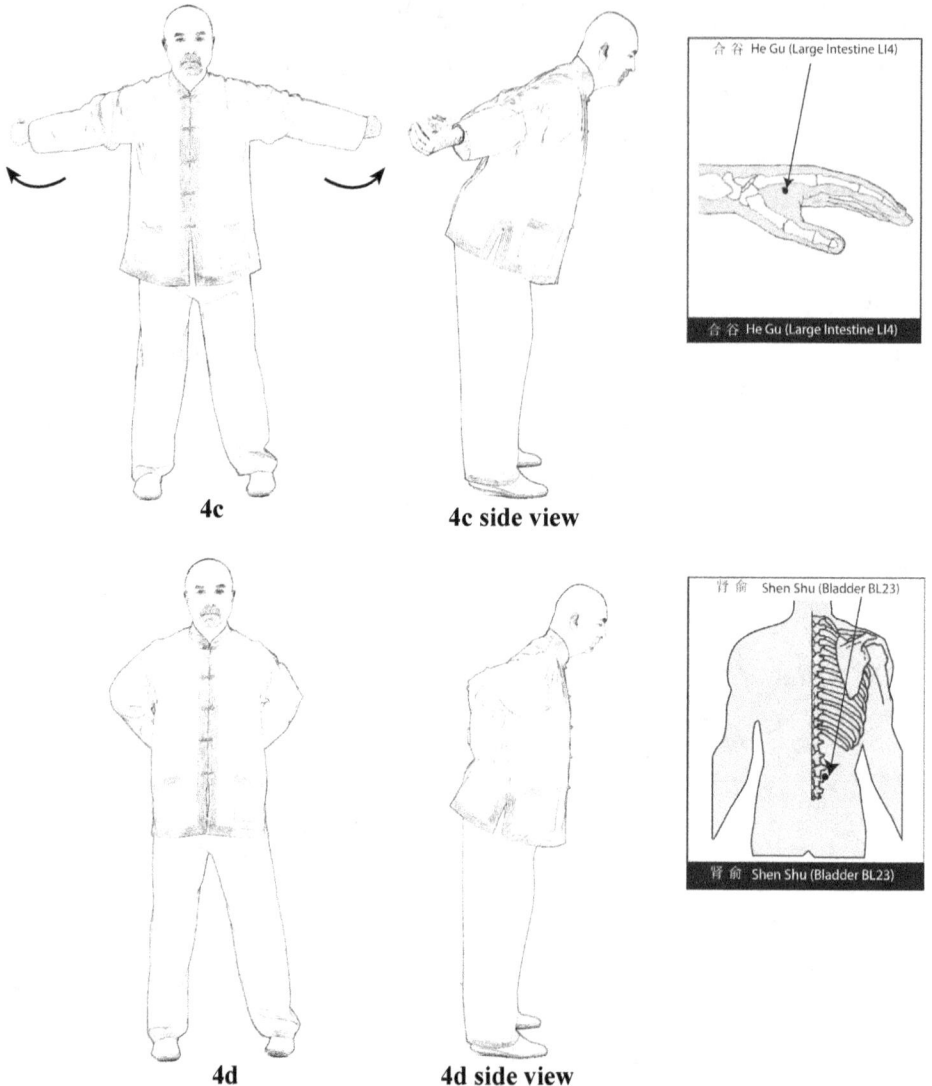

4c

4c side view

合谷 He Gu (Large Intestine LI4)

合谷 He Gu (Large Intestine LI4)

腎俞 Shen Shu (Bladder BL23)

腎俞 Shen Shu (Bladder BL23)

4d

4d side view

4b When they reach the height of your chest, push them out (palms facing outward) and lean forward 45°. At the same time, raise your heels off the ground and bring your bodyweight onto the balls of the feet.

This energetically connects the He Gu (web of hand) with the Qi Hu (beneath collar bone).

4c Slowly straighten your back and bring your arms around to the side of the body drawing four fingers together with the thumb to form the Plum Blossom Claw. At the same time, stand up higher on the toes.

4d Relax your shoulders and rotate the arms behind your body and touch the He Gu (web of hand) with Shen Shu (beneath the Kidneys).

5. Thrusting the wings forward 抖膀

These movements release the negative or stale Qi into the earth.

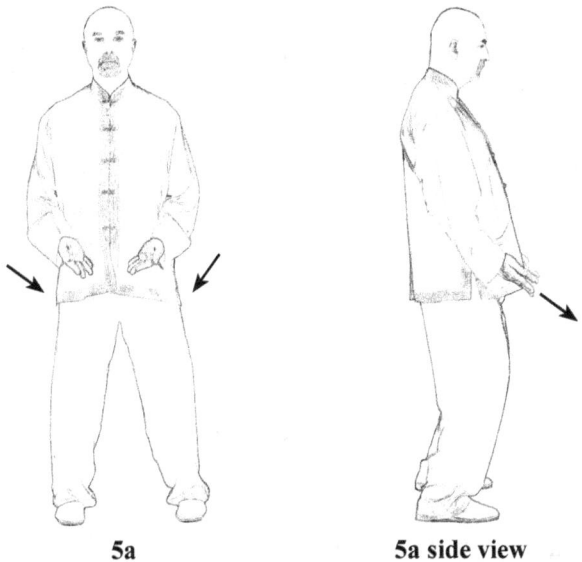

5a   **5a side view**

5a Relax your elbows and wrists and draw the hands around the waist (Belt Channel). Quickly flick the arms and thrust and release the Plum Blossom Claw forward, simultaneously dropping down on the heels. Your hands should be slightly turned in toward each other with the wrists lower than the elbows. The fingers are open and relaxed to release the stale Qi.

6. Drawing the wings to the back 折窝 (same as movement No. 4)

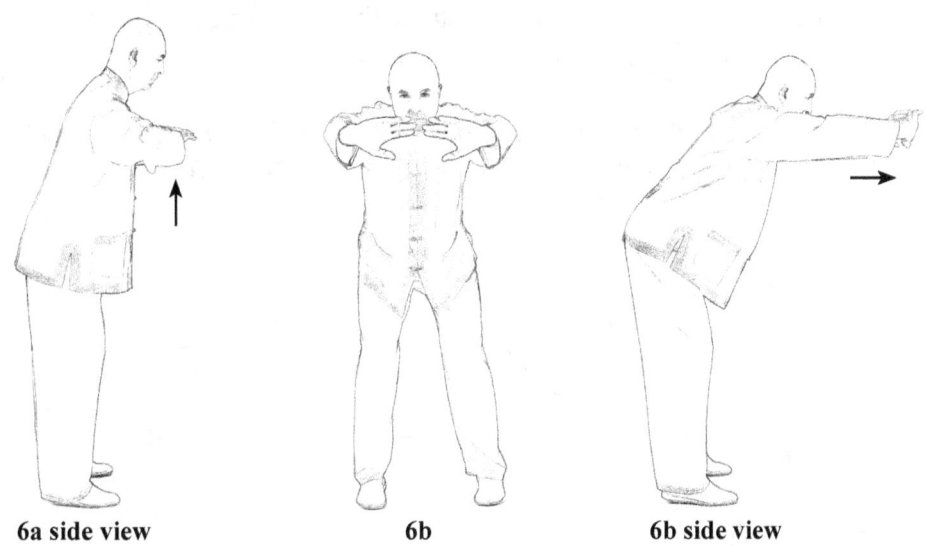

6a side view   **6b**   **6b side view**

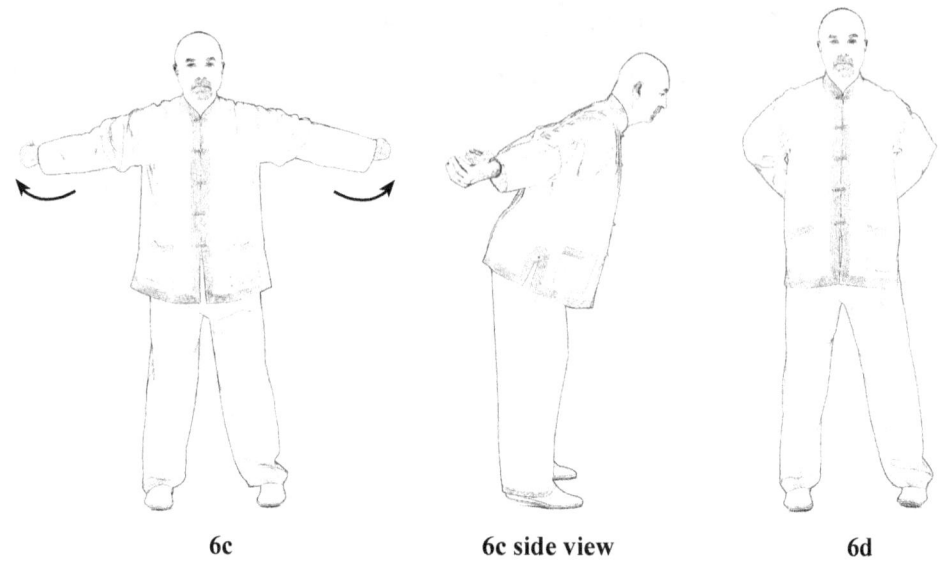

| 6c | 6c side view | 6d |

6a Gently straighten your back, lowering the heels to the ground. Your eyes are looking straight ahead. With a slight bend at the waist, slowly scoop the hands up in front of your body with the fingers pointing towards each other.

6b When they reach chest height push them out (palms facing outward) and lean forward 45°. At the same time, raise your heels off the ground and bring your bodyweight onto the balls of the feet.

6c Slowly straighten your back and bring your arms around to the side of the body drawing four fingers together with the thumb to form the Plum Blossom Claw. At the same time, stand up higher on the toes.

6d Relax your shoulders and rotate the arms behind the body and touch the He Gu (web of hand) with Shen Shu (beneath the Kidneys).

7. Thrusting the wings forward 抖膀 (same as movement No. 5)

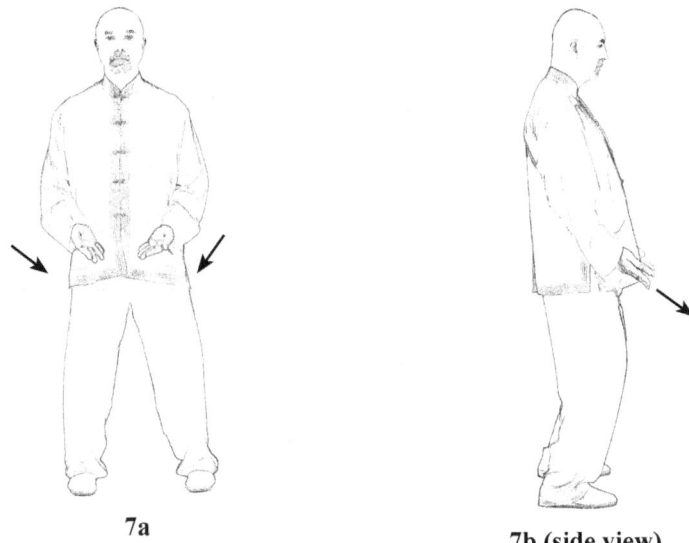

7a

7b (side view)

7a Relax your elbows and wrists and draw the hands around the waist (Dai Mai Channel). Quickly flick the arms and thrust and release the Plum Blossom Claw forward, simultaneously dropping down on the heels. The hands should be slightly turned in toward each other with the wrists lower than the elbows. Fingers are open and relaxed to release the negative or stale Qi.

8.   Lifting the wings 上举

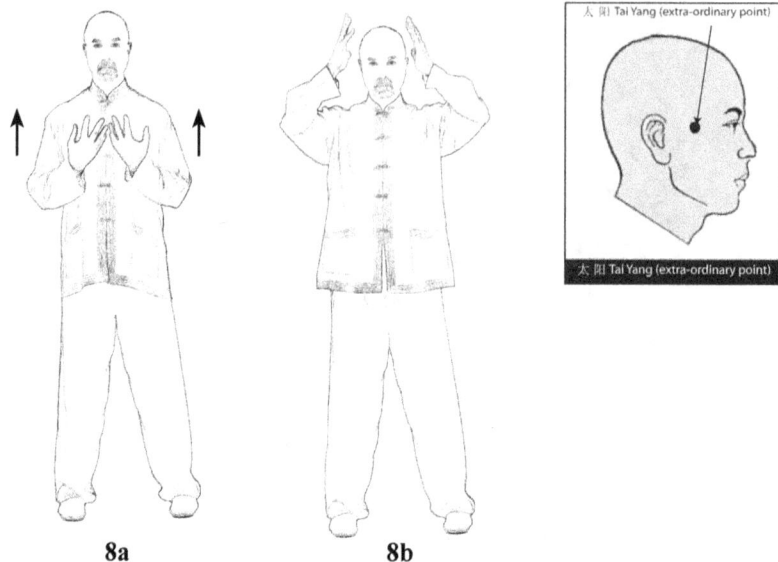

8a   8b

8a   Keeping your shoulders relaxed, scoop hands up and raise arms with palms facing the body and the fingers pointing towards the sky. Raise hands to your forehead looking at the Lao Gong (middle of palm).

8b   Hands circle around to the side of the face connecting the Lao Gong (middle of palm) with the Tai Yang (extra-ordinary point) located at the temple, 3cm back from the eyes.

9.　Interlocking the wings 合掌

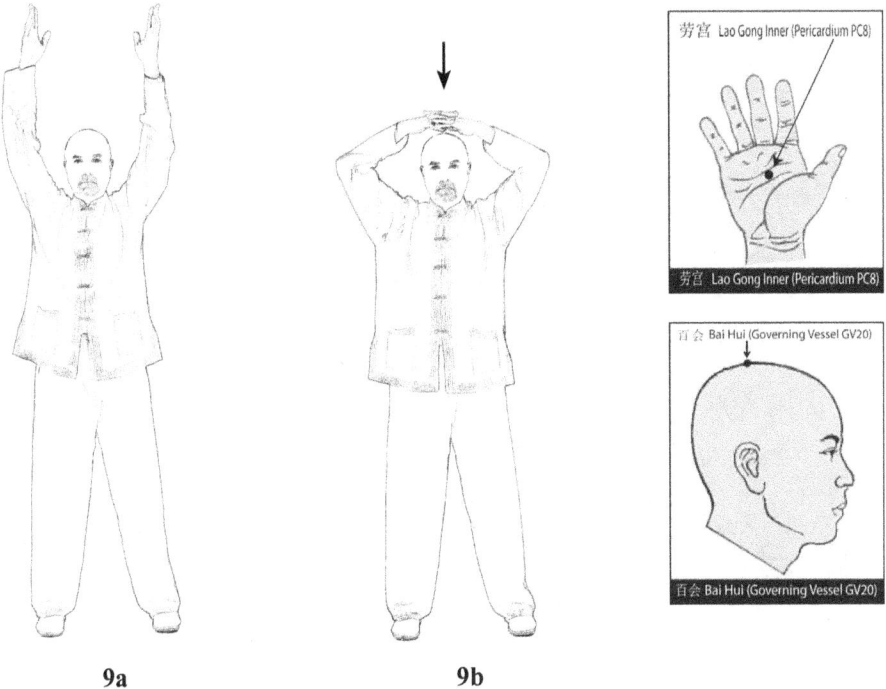

9a   9b

9a Lift your arms above your head, with the palms facing each other.

9b Relax your wrists and turn your palms to top of your head. Interlock the fingers and lower the hands. The Lao Gong (middle of palm) connects to the Bai Hui (Governing Vessel GV20) at the top of the head translating to a hundred points converge. Imagine a line lengthwise from your nose to the top of your head connecting with a line from the tip of your ears, converging at the top and middle of your head.

10.   Turning the palms up 翻掌

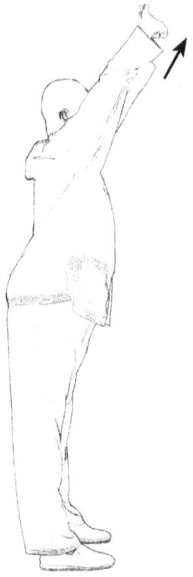

10a side view

10a   Turn your palms out, keeping the fingers interlocked. Slowly straighten your arms while looking at the palms. Gently stretch the arms, back and legs.

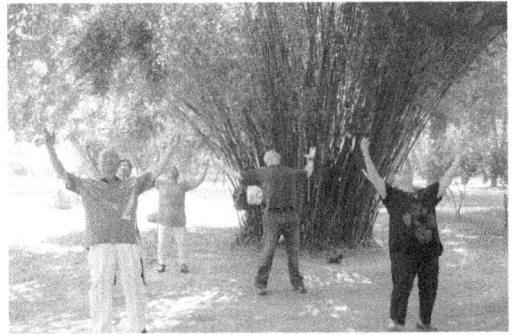

Spreading the wings 展翅

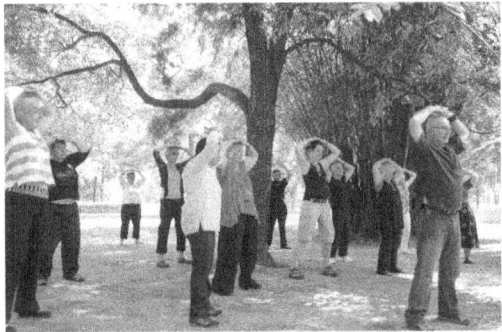

Interlocking the wings 合掌

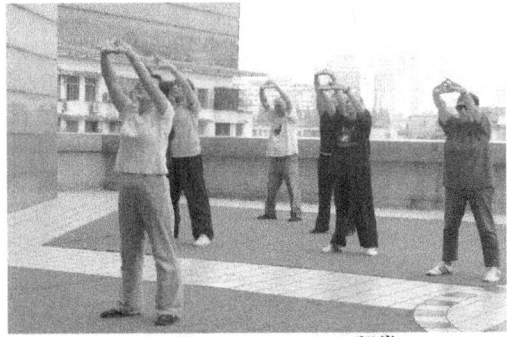

Turning the palms up 翻掌

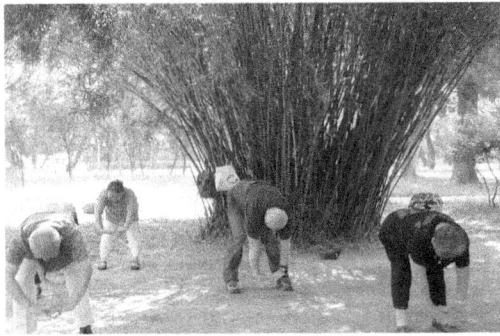

Bending the waist 下腰

11. Bending the waist 下腰

It is important to keep your legs straight when bending forward as these movements stimulate the Kidney Channels and help strengthen the back and waist area.

The First 11 Movements
This set of 11 movements can be practised as an isolated set of movements. The sequence opens the Ren and Du Channels which benefits the Upper, Lower and Middle Dan Tian. The set of movements improves overall blood circulation of the body and benefits the vascular system and the Kidneys.

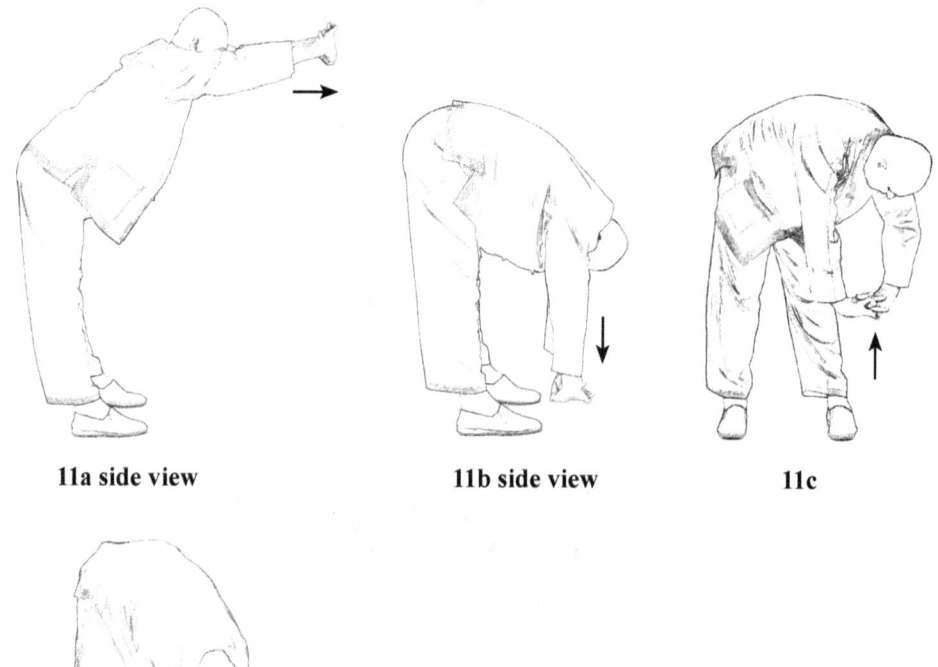

11a side view   11b side view   11c

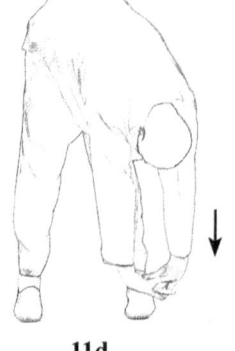

11d

11a Keeping the legs straight, gently push your bottom back as you stretch forward and bend from the waist.

11b Push your palms down to face the ground and stretch as far as you feel comfortable.

11c,d Lift the upper body and bend your arms slightly until your hands are about knee height; then push towards the left small toe. Stretch down as far as you feel comfortable.

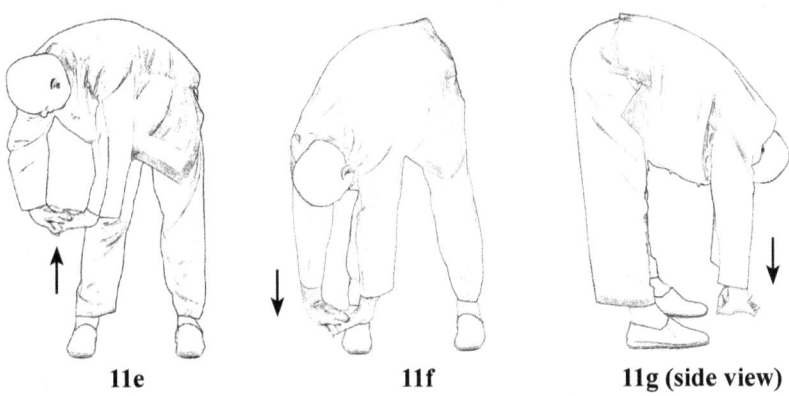

11e   **11f**   **11g (side view)**

11e,f   Lift your upper body and arms again to knee height and stretch down to the right small toe.

11g   Lift your upper body and repeat the stretch to the centre.

It is important to do these movements gently to start with and only stretch as far as you feel comfortable. With regular practice your level of flexibility and strength will increase.

12. Twining the hands 缠手

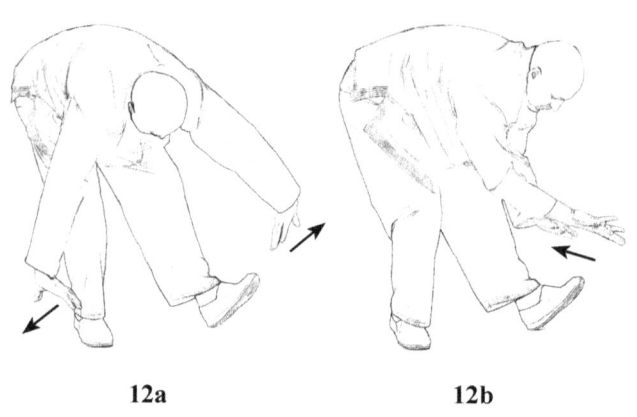

12a   **12b**

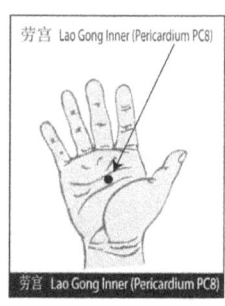

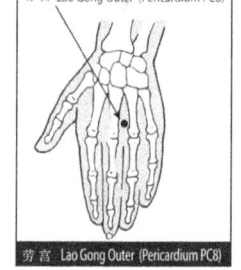

12a   Bend your knees slightly and simultaneously move your bodyweight to the right foot pivoting on the left heel and lifting your left toes up to point to the sky. At the same time, separate your hands with the palms facing the ground, and, with the elbows relaxed, move your arms in a circular shape. The He Gu (web of hand) and fingers of both hands are facing each other, and your finger tips are over the tip of the toes. This movement is performed quickly in one motion.

12b   Keeping your bodyweight over the right leg, turn from the waist and move your right arm to the left, in the Southern direction. Keep you wrists, hands and fingers relaxed as if the back of the fingers are paint brush bristles making a line on the earth. When the right elbow is over the left hand, turn both palms up. The left palm should be about 2cm under the right elbow. From this position and moving from the waist, draw your right arm back so that the Inner Lao Gong (middle of palm) of the left hand can energetically cross the Outer Lao Gong (middle of hand) of the right hand. This movement is a spiralling action similar to twining two pieces of rope together.

13. Recovering the Qi 回气

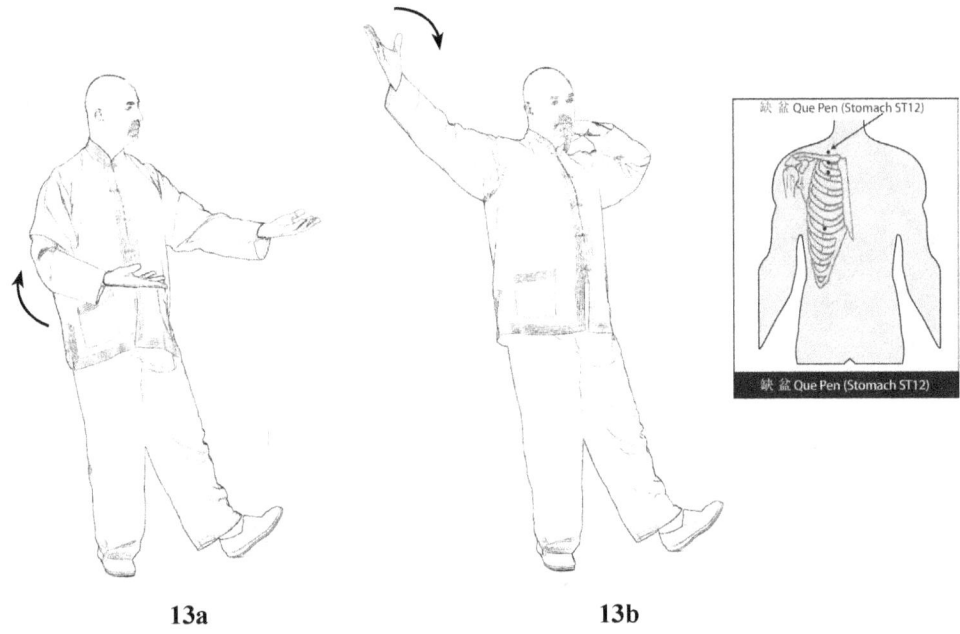

13a   13b

13a   Keeping your bodyweight over the right leg and left toes pointing to the sky, gently lift your upper body and the arms; the arms rise with the body. Relax your arms and shoulders with palms facing up.

13b   Turning from the waist, your right arms swings to the right. Your chest is facing the Southern direction and your right hand is facing the Northern direction. Bend the left elbow, form the Plum Blossom Claw (four fingers touching together with the thumb) and touch the left Que Pen (Stomach ST12) the indentation above the middle of the collar bone.

14. Twisting the left toes 左弹足

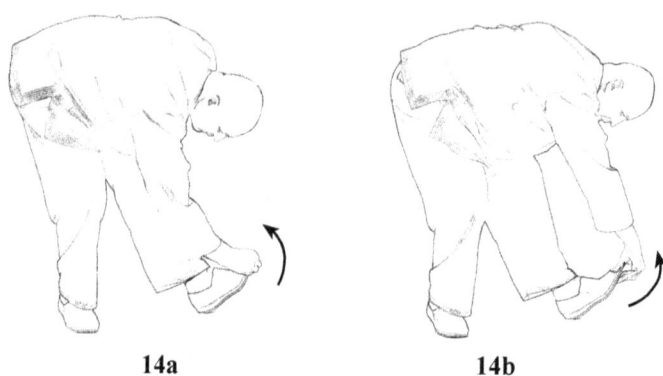

14a   14b

14a   With your bodyweight over the right leg and the left toes pointing to the sky, continue to swing your right arm up. When it is over your head bend from the waist and place the right thumb between the big toe and the second toe and wrap your fingers around the bottom of the foot. This stimulates both the Spleen and Liver channels which originate from this area.

14b   With a slightly bent elbow move the upper body three times in a circular anti-clockwise direction from the waist by pressing the right elbow and shoulder outwards from the body.

This movement should be done gently without too much strain on the body. If your flexibility does not allow you to touch your toes, the right fingers can point toward the left big toe. With the elbow slightly bent, make the same three anti-clockwise movements with the upper body.

Benefit: This movement aids the digestive system by twisting and stimulating the Spleen area.

15. Pushing away the Qi 推气

In this movement the hand draws an oval shape, scanning, feeling and receiving Qi from the earth.

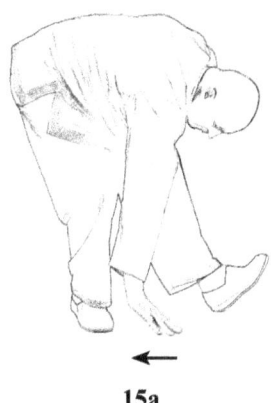

15a

15a   Keep your bodyweight over the right leg, point left toes to the sky and keep the left Plum Blossom Claw (four fingers touching together with the thumb) touching the left Que Pen (above the collar bone). Relax the right hand with the palm facing the ground.

16. Scooping up the Qi 捞气

The scooping movement gathers the earth Qi which then connects with the Que Pen (above collar bone) to stimulate the Stomach Channel and send the energy down.

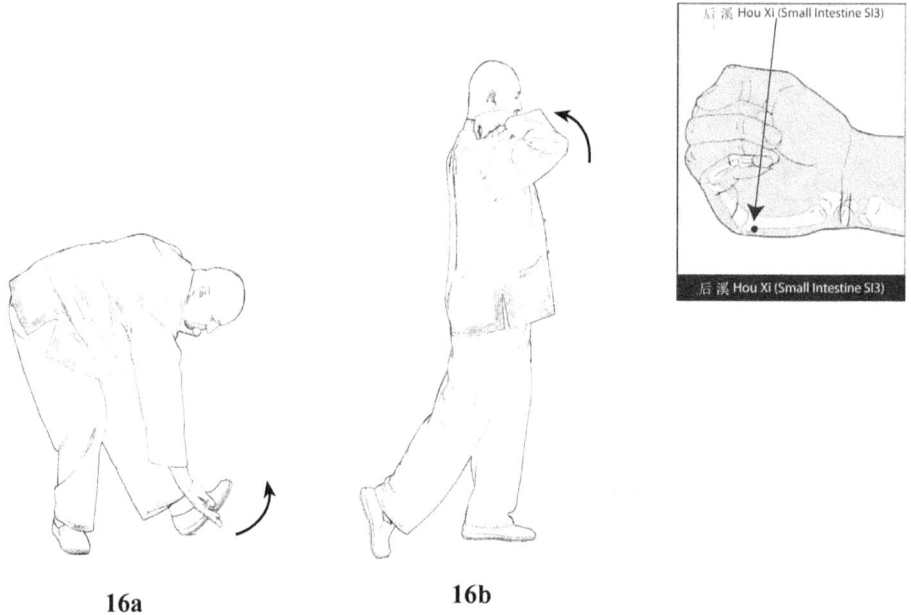

16a   16b

16a   When your right hand circles behind your right foot, turn the palm up to face the sky, scooping up the Qi and moving your bodyweight forward. This is similar to drawing the letter 'b' on the earth.

16b   The left arm remains unchanged, with the left Plum Blossom Claw (four fingers touching together with the thumb) touching the left Que Pen (above the collar bone). The point on the side of the hand, the Hou Xi (Small Intestine S13) gently touches the neck beneath the ear. As your bodyweight moves forward over the left leg your right hand forms the Plum Blossom Claw and touches the right Que Pen (beneath collar bone) and the Hou Xi (edge of hand) near the neck. Hips, shoulders and elbows are pointing straight ahead facing the Southern direction and all your bodyweight is on the left leg and the right heel is off the ground.

17. Turning the body and recovering the Qi 转身回气

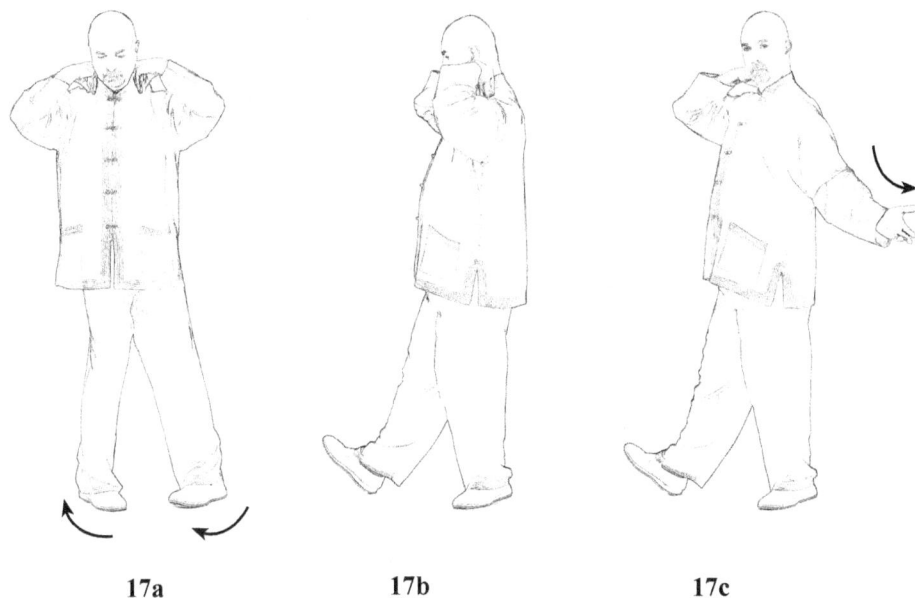

17a   17b   17c

17a   Move your bodyweight back to the right leg and turn your left foot to the right and hook it around as far as feels comfortable.

17b   Move your bodyweight back to the left leg and pivot on the right heel lifting your right toe to face the sky. The hips and shoulders are facing the Northern direction and all your bodyweight is on the left leg.

17c   Release the left Plum Blossom Claw and lower your arm in front of your body, palm facing to the sky. Turning from the waist, the left arm swings to the left whilst looking at your left hand.

18. Twisting the right toes 右弹足

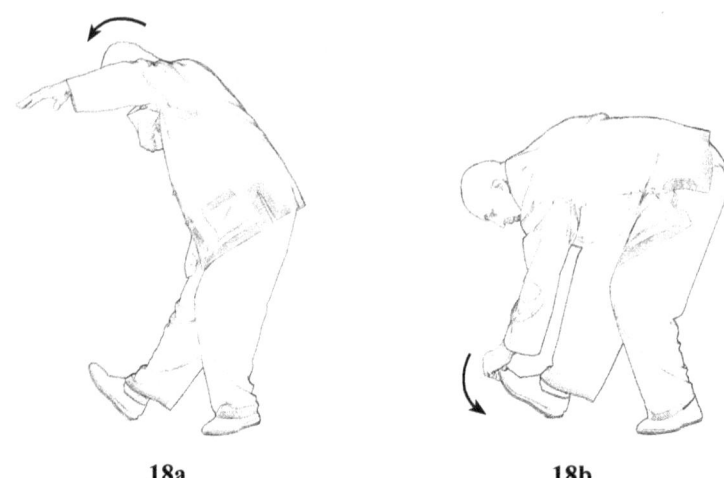

18a   18b

18a   Keeping your bodyweight over the left leg and right toes pointing to the sky, swing your left arm up and when it is over your head bend from the waist and place the left thumb between the big toe and the second toe and wrap your fingers around the bottom of the foot. This stimulates both the Spleen and Liver channels which originate from this area.

18b   With a slightly bent elbow move the upper body three times in a circular anti-clockwise direction from the waist by pressing the left elbow outwards from the body.

This movement is the same as movement no. 14, but to the other side. Importantly, it should be done gently without too much strain on the body. If your flexibility does not allow you to touch your toes, the left fingers can point toward the right big toe. With the elbow slightly bent, make the same three anti-clockwise movements with the upper body.

Benefit: This movement improves Liver function by twisting and stimulating the Liver area.

19. Pushing away the Qi 推气

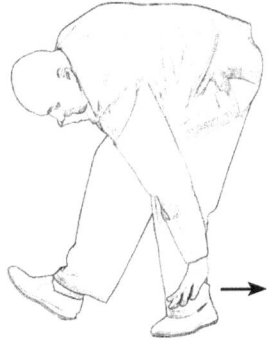

w19a With your bodyweight over the left leg, right toes pointing to the sky, and the right Plum Blossom Claw touching the right Que Pen (above the collar bone), relax the left hand with the palm facing the ground. The hand draws an oval shape, scanning, feeling and receiving Qi from the earth.

20. Scooping up the Qi 捞气

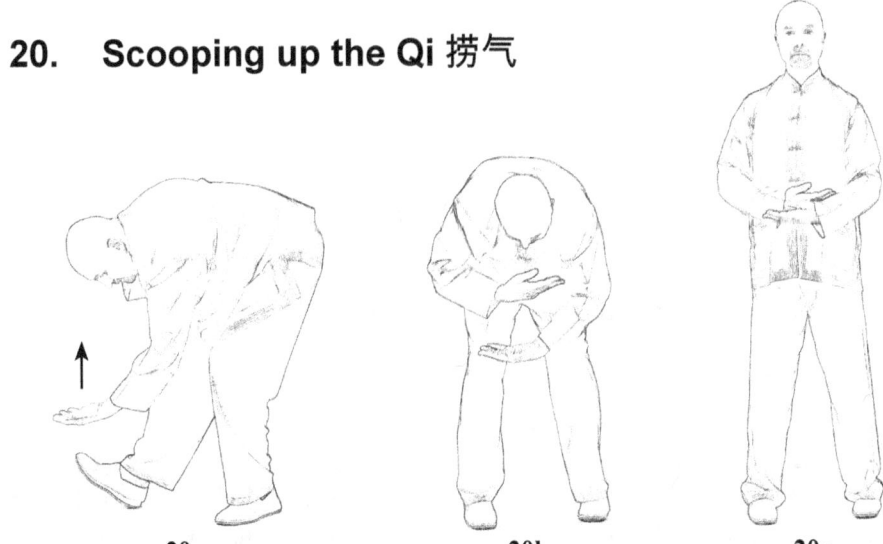

| 20a | 20b | 20c |

20a When your left hand circles behind the left foot turn your palm up to face the sky and scoop up the Qi.

20b Pivot on your right heel and turn the toe to face the Western direction. Adjust left foot so both feet are parallel. Release the right Plum Blossom Claw, palms facing the sky.

20c Slowly straighten your back lifting your upper body from the waist. Looking at your hands, move your right palm down to meet the left palm in front of your waist. When your body is fully upright, your eyes will be looking straight ahead.

21. Rotating the hands 缠手

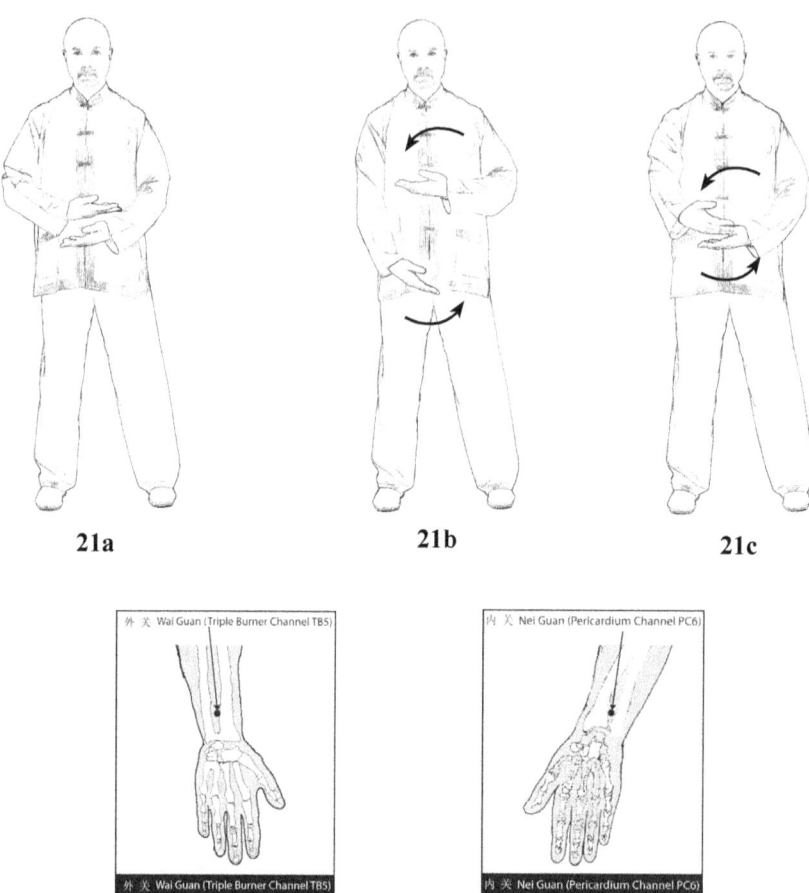

21a   21b   21c

外 关 Wai Guan (Triple Burner Channel TB5)

内 关 Nei Guan (Pericardium Channel PC6)

21a,b,c   With the right hand moving up on the inside of the left hand, and the left hand moving down over the right hand, continue to rotate the hands in a circular motion. Rotate one and a half turns with each hand at about 3cm apart. Two points rotate around each other - the Nei Guan (Pericardium Channel PC6) in the middle of the <u>inner</u> arm between the two bones, about 5cm from the wrist, and the Wai Guan (Triple Burner Channel TB5) which is directly opposite on the <u>outer</u> arm between the two bones about 5cm from the wrist. Look at your hands while they are rotating.

Benefit: This movement helps regulate the Stomach Channels.

22. Cloud hands 云手

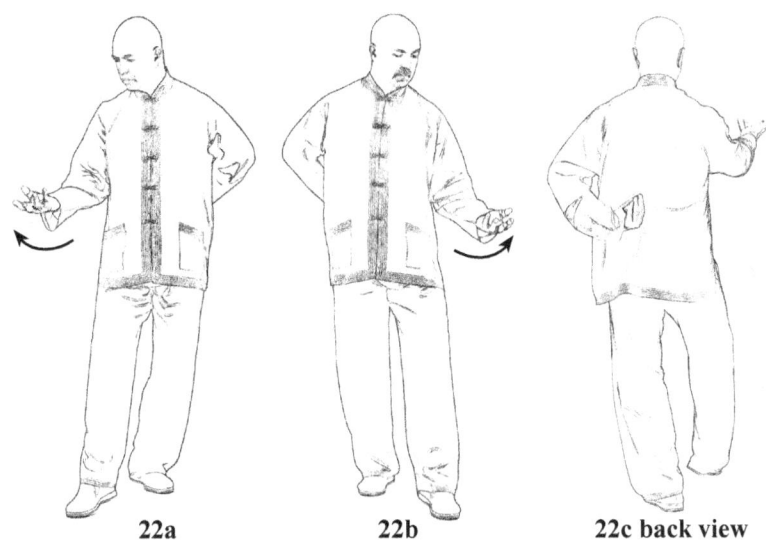

22a 22b 22c back view

22a   Relax your left arm with the left palm facing up (turning a little inward) and resting on your left hip at the waist on the Dai Mai. Keeping your weight on the left leg place your right foot forward half a step in front with only the outer edge of the foot (small toe) touching. As the same time, move your right arm forward with your palm turned up at waist height; your eyes are looking straight ahead. Turning from the waist, your eyes follow the right hand as it circles forward and behind your body. The hand is soft and relaxed as if a lotus flower is resting in your palm (lotus palm). Relax the elbow as the He Gu (web of hand) gently touches the Shen Shu (beneath the Kidneys).

22b   Step forward and bring your bodyweight over the right leg and gently place the outer part of your left foot (small toe) half a step in front, only just touching. At the same time, move the left arm forward at waist height and turn from the waist with your eyes looking at the lotus palm. Your left arm circles forward and around behind your body; relax the elbow as the He Gu (web of hand) gently touches the Shen Shu (beneath the Kidneys).

22c   These movements are repeated gently and smoothly to each side, like moving hands in the clouds. There is a total of four half steps finishing with the right hand behind your back. These stepping movements are similar to a Dayan or great bird gently stepping forward.

Benefit: This movement is beneficial for eyesight and hearing.

23.　Twisting the waist 涮腰

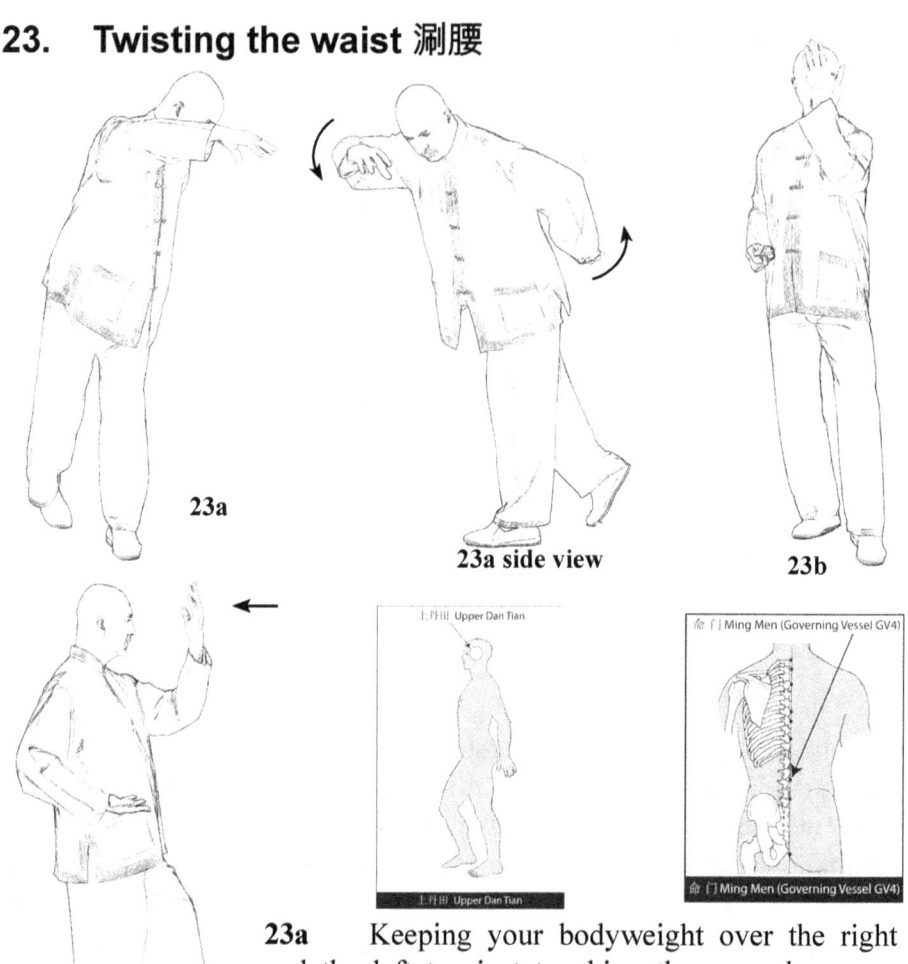

23a

23a side view

23b

23b side view

23a　Keeping your bodyweight over the right leg and the left toe just touching the ground, move your bodyweight forward onto the left leg twisting from the waist; your body turns so you are looking behind. This brings the right heel off the ground. At the same time, the right arm swings up and around with the He Gu (web of hand) facing towards the Upper Dan Tian (between the eyebrows), and the left arm swings behind with the He Gu (web of hand) facing towards the Ming Men (Governing Vessel GV4) on the lower back directly behind the navel.

23b　Quickly swing the upper body back, twisting from the waist. At the same time, move your bodyweight back onto the right leg, making a sharp, forceful stomping movement which grounds the weight onto the right heel. All your bodyweight is on the right leg with the left toe just touching the ground. The right arm swings down with the palm facing up and rests on the right waist; the left arm swings up with the Lao Gong (middle of palm) about 5cm from the Upper Dan Tian (between the eyebrows).

Benefit: This movement strengthens the back and helps regulate the digestive system.

24. Dropping the wings and recovering the Qi 落榜回气

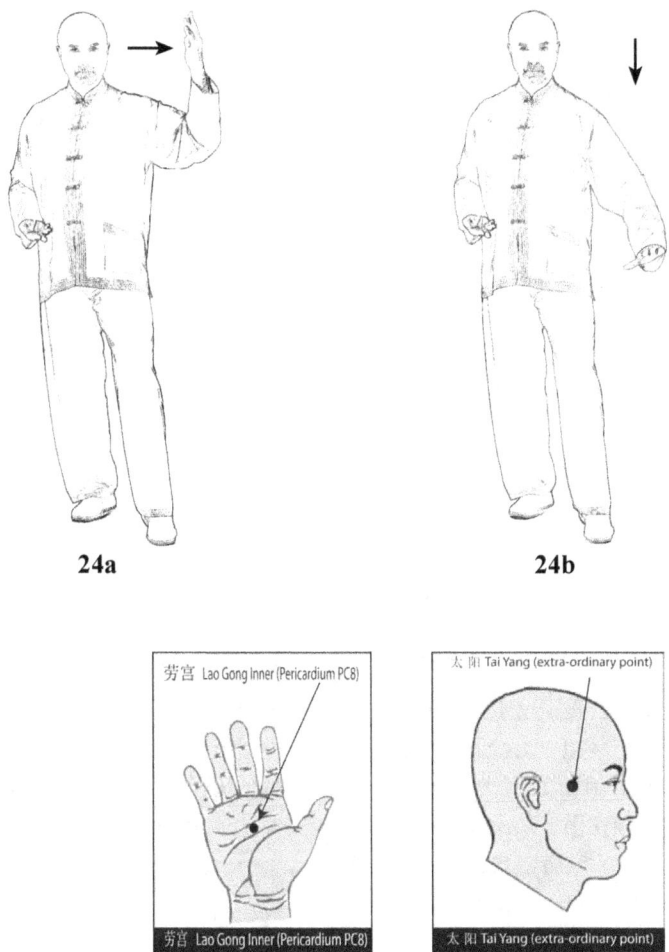

24a   24b

劳宫 Lao Gong Inner (Pericardium PC8)

太阳 Tai Yang (extra-ordinary point)

劳宫 Lao Gong Inner (Pericardium PC8)

太阳 Tai Yang (extra-ordinary point)

24a   Keeping your bodyweight over the right leg with the left toe just touching the ground, the left hand Lao Gong (middle of palm) traces around the front of your head to the Tai Yang located at the temple, 2cm from the side of the eye.

24b   With your left palm turning down, slowly lower your hand towards the side of the buttock. Keeping the elbow relaxed and arm curved, the palm faces the ground with your fingers pointing forward.

25. Lifting the single wing 单展翅

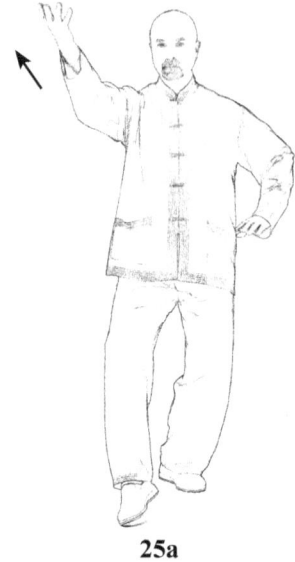

25a

25a   Move your bodyweight forward onto the left leg and take a small step with the right small toe just touching the ground. At the same time, your right arm moves forward in front of your face; eyes are looking straight ahead. Turning to the right from the waist your eyes follow the right hand as it circles around and behind your body. Relax the elbow as the He Gu (web of hand) gently touches the Shen Shu (beneath the Kidneys).

Benefit: This movement improves Kidneys function and helps regulate blood pressure.

26. Stepping forward and extending the wing 上步伸膀

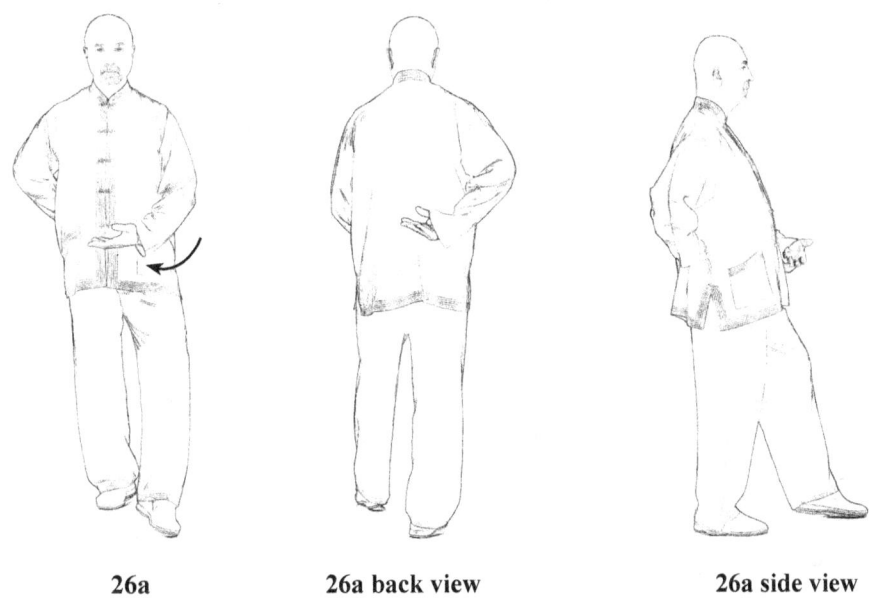

26a   **26a back view**   **26a side view**

26a   Move your bodyweight forward onto the right leg and take a small step forward with the left small toe just touching the ground. The left hands draws a circle in towards the body, keeping the shoulder and elbow relaxed. Turn your left palm up in front of the Lower Dan Tian (area beneath the navel). Look at the palm of your hand. The right hand stays connected to the Shen Shu (beneath the Kidneys).

27. Winding the hand around the head and the ears 缠头过耳

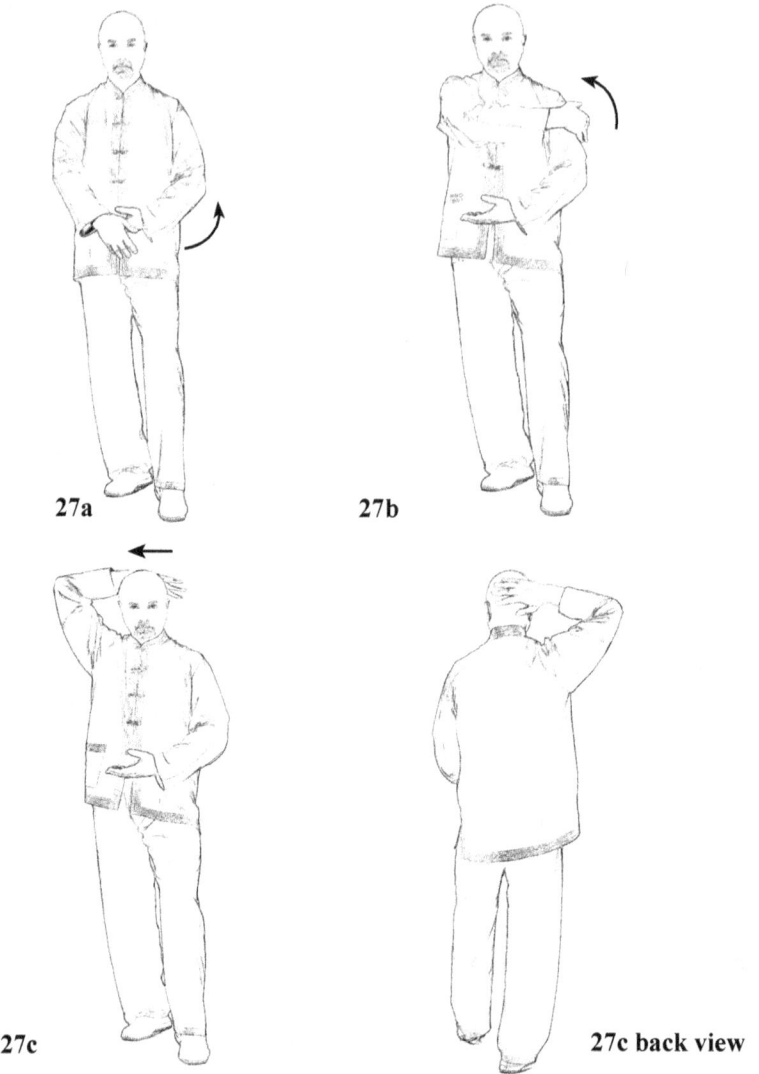

27a   27b

27c   27c back view

27a   Keeping your bodyweight over the right leg and the left small toe just touching the ground, turn from the waist and move your right arm in front of the abdomen.

27b,c   The Lao Gong (middle of palm) of the right hand traces around the outside of the left arm to the elbow, to the shoulder, around the left ear and across the back of the head to the right ear; the palm is now facing forward. Straighten your head and look forward, keeping shoulders and elbows relaxed.

Benefit: This movement is good for the eyesight as well as thyroid problems and hearing difficulties. For problems with high blood pressure move the right hand higher over the top of the head (Bai Hui).

28.   Pressing the Qi down 下压

This movement and the next movement are slow and smooth helping to harmonise and balance Yin and Yang by gathering and dispersing Qi from the earth.

The movements from 28 to 35 are for dispelling Yin and nurturing Yang energy. The more you do the exercises in this section, the more you process and gather pure Qi into the Lower Dan Tian (area beneath the navel) for healing purposes.

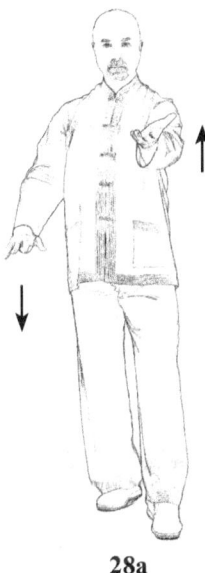

28a   With your bodyweight in the same position, move the right arm down in front of your body with the palm facing the earth, and at the same time move the left arm up in front of the body with the palm facing the sky. The right hand descends to the hip area and the left hand rises to the forehead.

28a

29.   Pulling the Qi up 上托

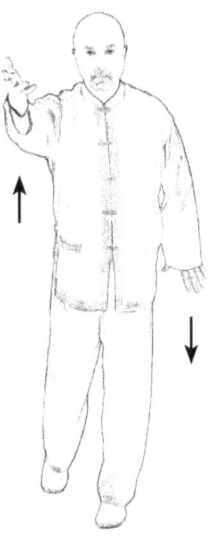

29a   Reverse the position of your hands by turning the right hand up to face the sky and the left hand to face the earth. Move your bodyweight forward onto the left leg as you raise the right arm forward and the left arm down. Bring all your bodyweight onto the left leg, lifting the right heel. The right arm rises to the height of your forehead and the left arm descends to the hip area.

29a

30.   Recovering the Qi 回气

The stomping in this movement is important as it collects and gathers Qi. This completes a process that receives, processes, disperses and formulates the Qi. Over time, with regular practice, these movements purify and refine Qi.

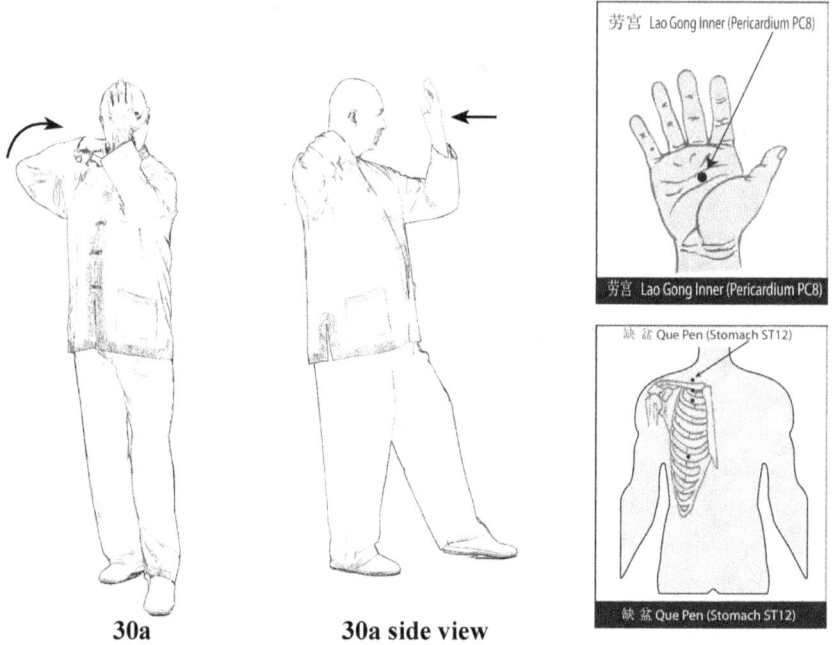

劳宫 Lao Gong Inner (Pericardium PC8)

劳宫 Lao Gong Inner (Pericardium PC8)

缺 盆 Que Pen (Stomach ST12)

缺 盆 Que Pen (Stomach ST12)

30a   **30a side view**

30a   Quickly thrust your left arm up and your right arm down as you move your bodyweight back onto the right leg, making a sharp stomping and forceful movement, grounding the weight onto the right heel. All your bodyweight is on the right leg with the left toe just touching the ground. The left arm swings up with the Lao Gong (middle of palm) pushing Qi into the Upper Dan Tian (between the eyebrows), while the right arm swings back with the right Plum Blossom Claw (four fingers touching together with the thumb) touching the right Que Pen (above the collar bone).

Benefit: The vibration caused by dropping the heel is good for the brain and for stimulating Qi toward to Upper Dan Tian.

31. Scooping the moon 捞月

The movements from 31 to 35 gather the Yin energy to stimulate and strengthen our Yin energy field.

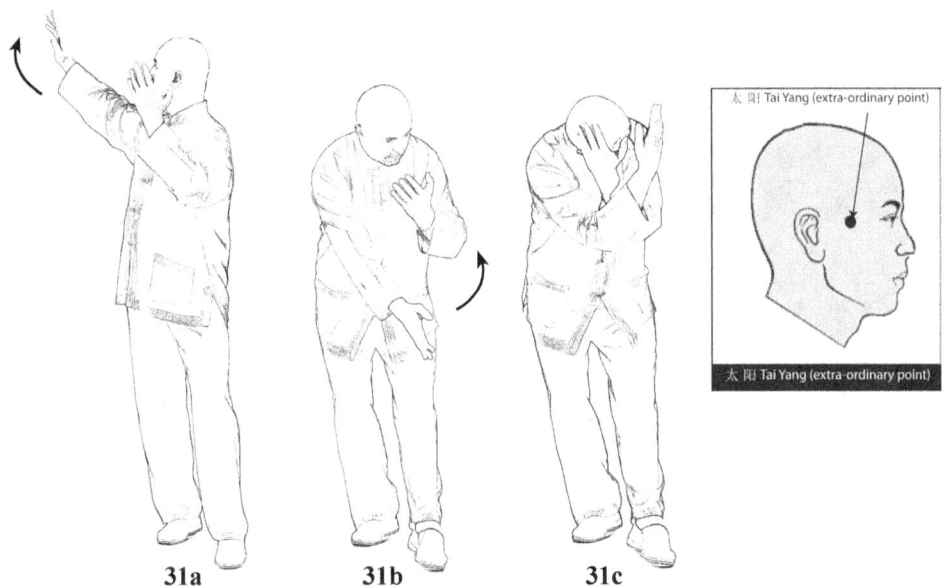

31a   31b   31c

31a   With your bodyweight over the right leg, the left small toe just touching the ground, and the left hand in front of the face, release the right Plum Blossom Claw (four fingers touching together with the thumb). With a relaxed right shoulder, elbow and hand, turn from the waist and scoop the right hand out to the North East direction.

31b   Turning from the waist, the right arm sweeps in front of the abdomen around to the left while at the same time bending forward from the waist.

31c   Crouching forward slightly from the waist with the upper body at an angle of about 45°, twist your body to the South West direction. The arms cross in front of your chest with the left arm on the inside and the Lao Gong (middle of palm) facing the right Tai Yang at the temple, 2cm to the side of the eye. Your right arm is on the outside with the Lao Gong (middle of palm) facing the Upper Dan Tian (between the eyebrows).

32. Turning around 转身

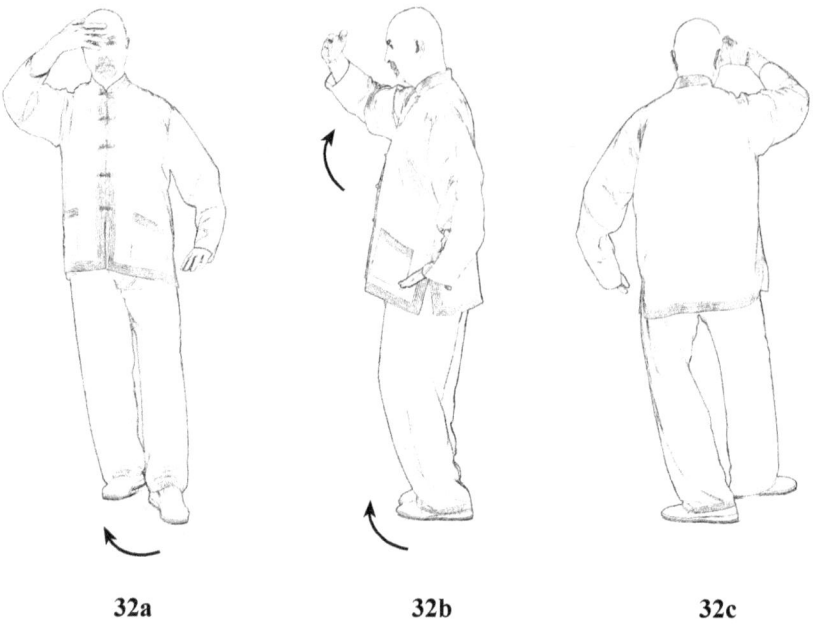

32a   32b   32c

32a   Slowly straighten your back by lifting the upper body. Continue to face the Western direction. Keeping your shoulder relaxed, straighten your left elbow and move your left hand down in front of the body and to the side of your left hip. Your left palm is facing the earth with your fingers pointing forward. Look at your right hand which is facing the Upper Dan Tian (between the eyebrows).

32b   Turn your body 180° to face the Eastern direction: move your bodyweight back onto the right leg and lift the left toes and turn to the right while pivoting on the left heel. Hook in the left toes as far as feels comfortable. Bend your knees slightly to avoid twisting and hurting your knees. The left toes are facing the North East direction.

32c   Move your bodyweight back onto the left leg and pivot on the right heel turning the right toes to the South East direction. Your body has turned 180° to face the Eastern direction.

33.　Stepping forward and looking at the palm 上步望掌

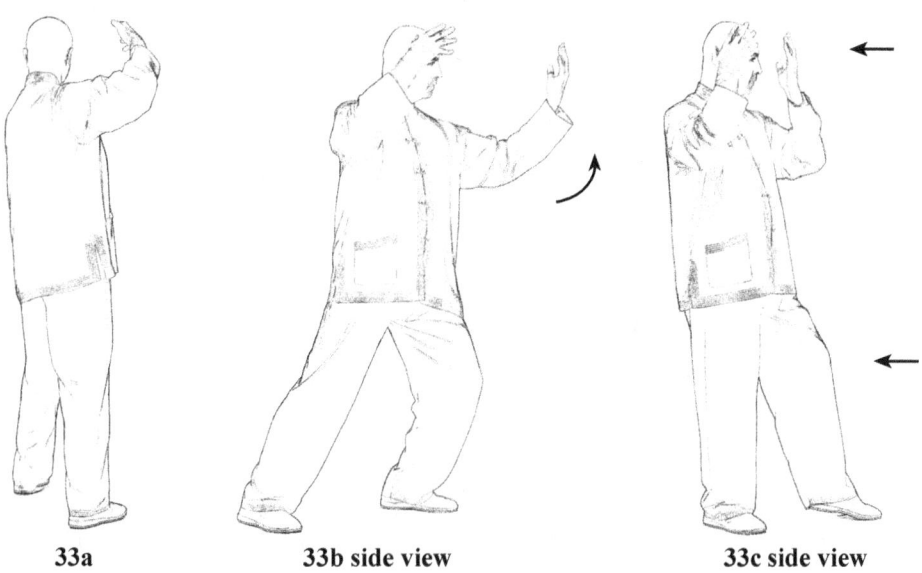

33a　　　　　　33b side view　　　　　33c side view

33a,b Gently move your bodyweight forward over the right leg and step forward with your left leg. The left toes are facing the Eastern direction with about 60% of your weight over the left leg. The right leg maintains about 40% of your weight with the heels and toes firmly grounded to the earth. At the same time that you transfer your bodyweight forward, the left arm moves forward with the body and the hand scoops up in front of the left waist, above the left foot.

33c Slowly move your bodyweight back onto the right leg with the left toes just touching the ground. At the same time, raise your left arm so the Lao Gong (middle of palm) pushes Qi into the Upper Dan Tian (between the eyebrows). Your right arm moves slightly to the right with the Lao Gong (middle of palm) facing the right Tai Yang (temple area).

34. Looking at the moon 望月

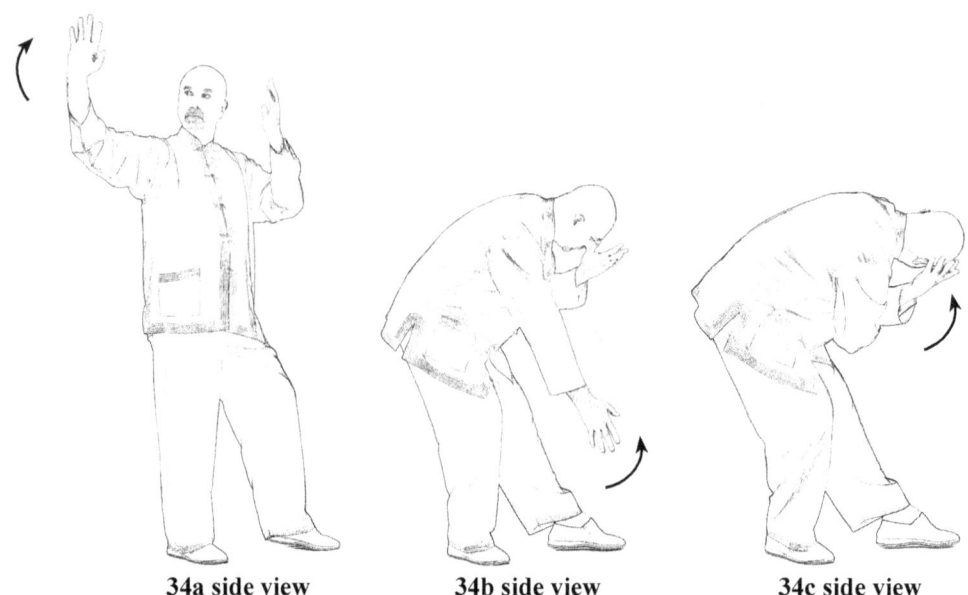

34a side view   34b side view   34c side view

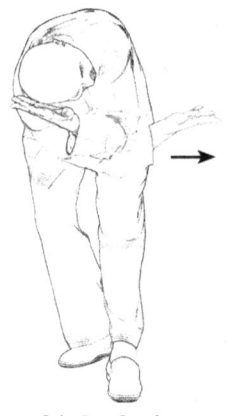

34c back view

34a Keep your bodyweight over the right leg with the left toes just touching the ground. The left hand is kept in front of your face and your shoulder, elbow and hand are relaxed. Turning from the waist, scoop your right hand out to the South West direction.

34b Your right arm sweeps down and around to the left whilst at the same time bending forward from the waist. Your right hand passes in front of the abdomen.

34c Crouching forward from the waist with the upper body at an angle slightly lower than 45°, twist the body slightly, looking to the Northern direction. The arms cross in front of your chest with the left arm on the inside and Lao Gong (middle of palm) facing the right Tai Yang (at the temple). The right arm sweeps around the outside with the inside of the right elbow touching the outside of the left elbow. The right hand finishes with a quick flicking movement with the eyes and fingers pointing to the Northern direction.

35.   Pressing the Qi 压气

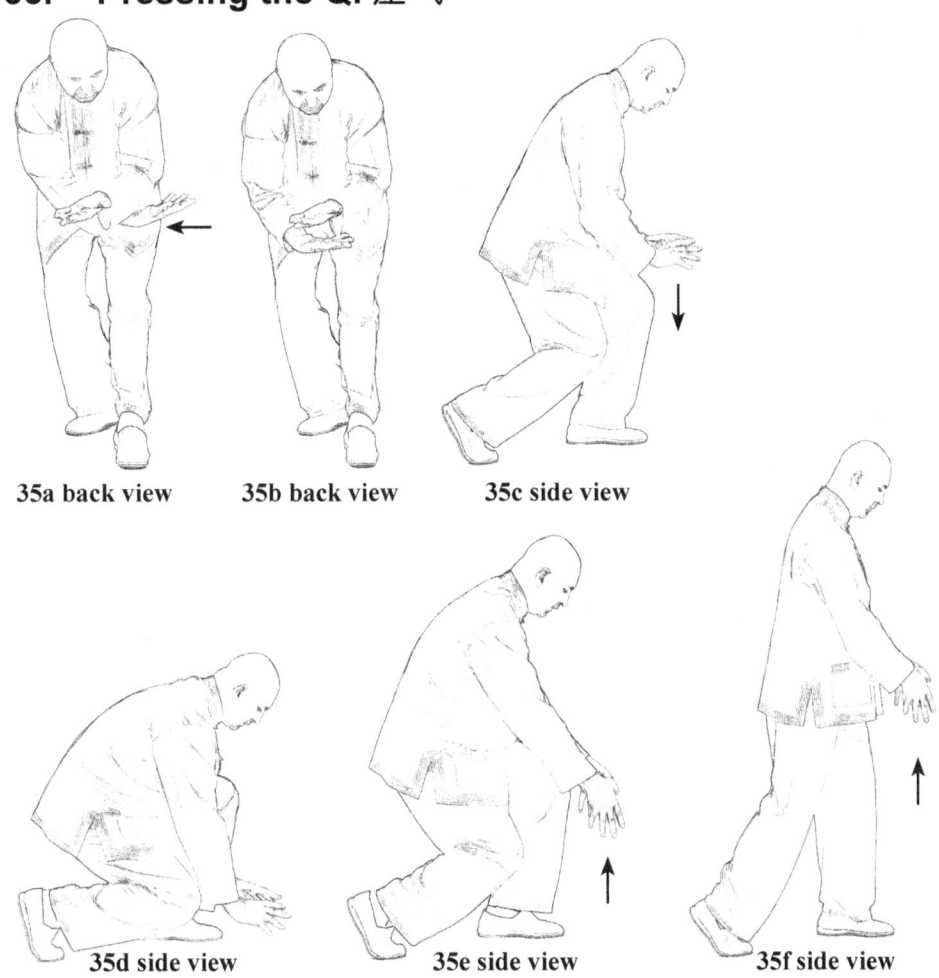

35a back view   35b back view   35c side view

35d side view   35e side view   35f side view

35a,b   Keeping your bodyweight over the right leg with the left toes just touching the ground, gently lift your upper body from the waist, keeping the shoulders and chest relaxed. Draw your right arm back slightly with the right palm moving under the left elbow.

35c   Take a half step forward with the left leg; at the same time, the right palm moves down on the outside of the left arm to the wrist and your back straightens to lift the upper body slightly.

35d   Move all of your bodyweight over the left leg and bend from the knee keeping the right toe just touching the ground. Look between your hands; the fingers face each other and are soft and relaxed as if holding a large egg. Gently press the earth in front of your left foot.

35e,f   Straighten the left leg to raise your body. Look at the hands, keeping fingers pointing towards the ground and separated and relaxed as if still holding an egg, and draw up the energy from the earth. The fingers are slightly tense.

Repeat three times.

36. Turning around and pressing the Qi 转身压气

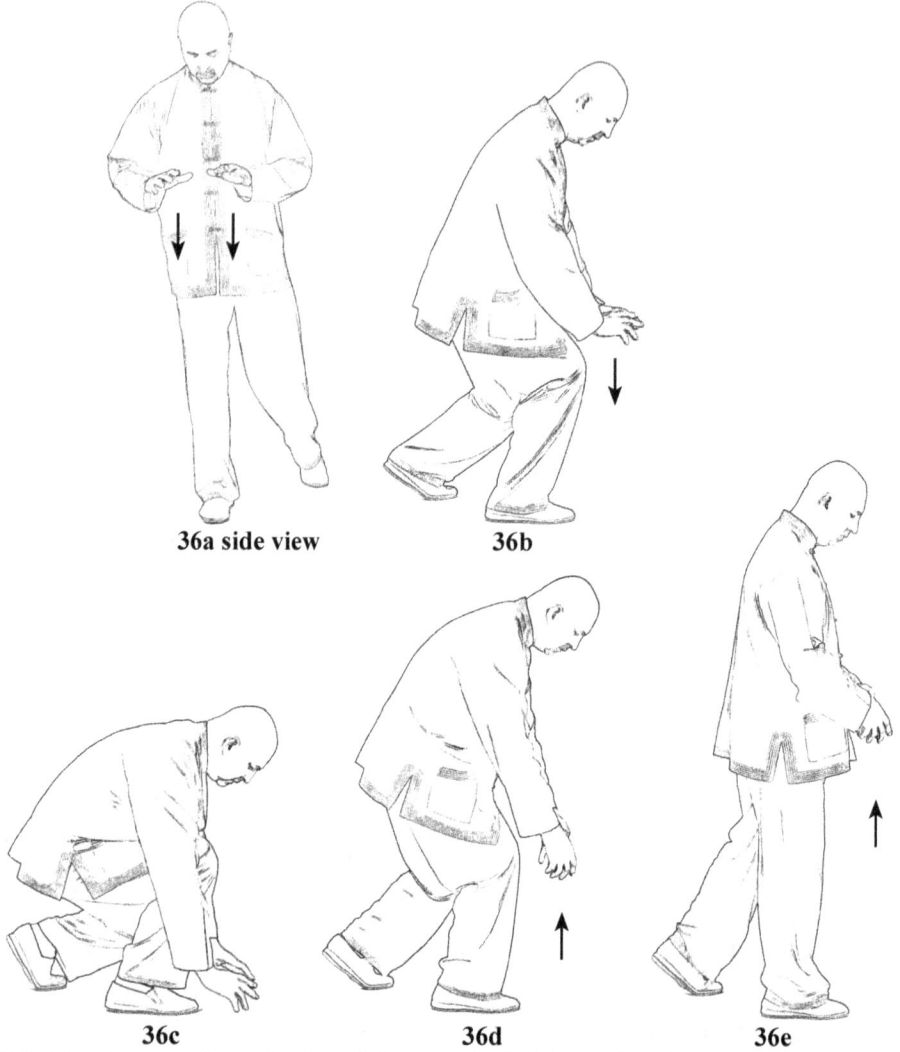

36a side view   **36b**

36c   **36d**   **36e**

36a Keeping all of your bodyweight over the left leg, raise the body and stand upright with your hands holding the 'egg' in front of the waist and palms facing the ground. Turn the right toe out 90° to face the Southern direction moving your bodyweight over the right leg and stepping behind with the left toe just touching the ground.

36b,c Keeping your bodyweight over the right leg, bend from the knees with the left toe just touching the ground. Look between your hands; the fingers face each other and are soft and relaxed as if holding a large egg. Gently press the earth in front of your right foot.

36d,e Straighten your right leg to raise the body. Look at the hands, keeping fingers pointing towards the ground and separated and relaxed as if still holding an egg, and draw up the energy from the earth. The fingers are slightly tense.

Repeat three times.

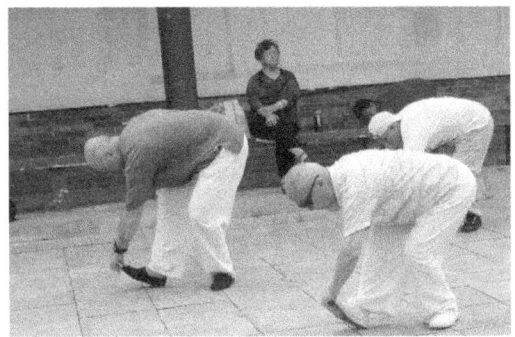

Twisting the right toes 右弹足

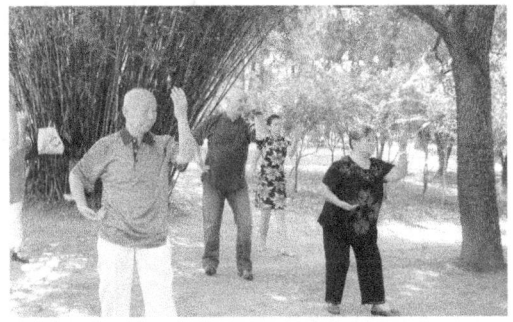

Dropping the wings and recover Qi   落榜回气

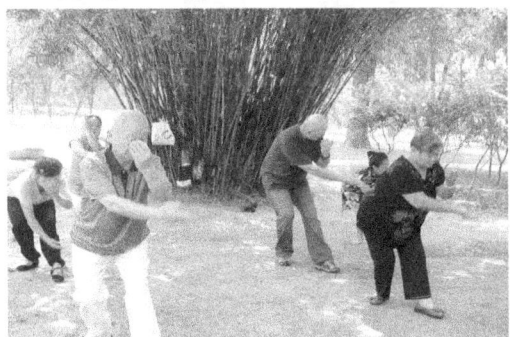

Looking at the moon   望月

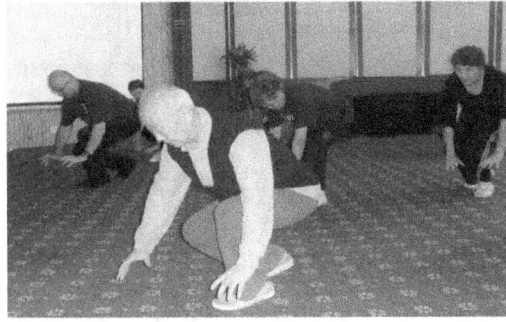

Pressing the Qi 压气

37.   Fluttering the wings 泳动

All the fluttering movements from 37 to 39 absorb the Qi into the Dai Mai belt and can benefit the Kidneys and Gall Bladder. The amplitude of the quiver is small and the frequency of it is high as this helps stimulate Qi through the whole body.

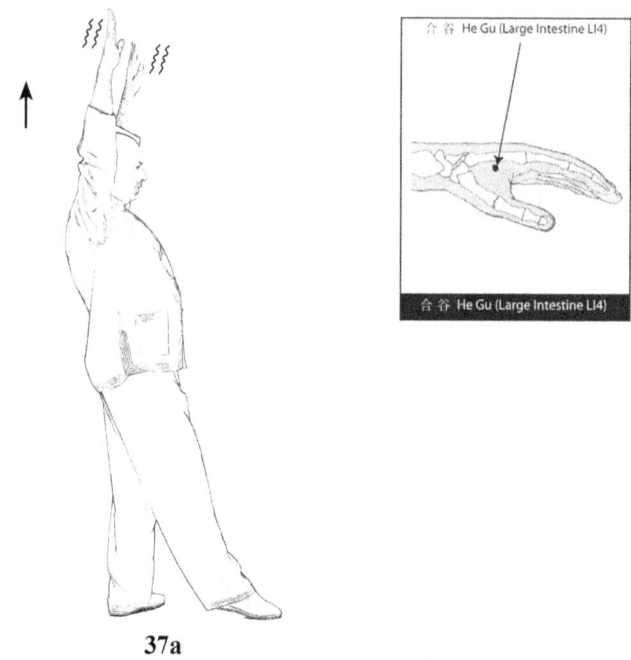

37a

37a   Straighten your right leg and raise the body; continue to look at your hands. Quiver or gently shake both hands and arms, similar to a bird fluttering its wings.

Move your bodyweight back onto the left leg and lift the right heel with the right toe just touching the ground. At the same time, raise the fluttering wings up overhead with the palms forward and fingers to the sky. The He Gu (web of hand) of both hands are facing each other. Keep your shoulders and elbows relaxed and arms about shoulder-width apart. With your eyes looking straight ahead stay in this position sensing the Qi for three seconds.

38.　Looking down at the water 瞰水

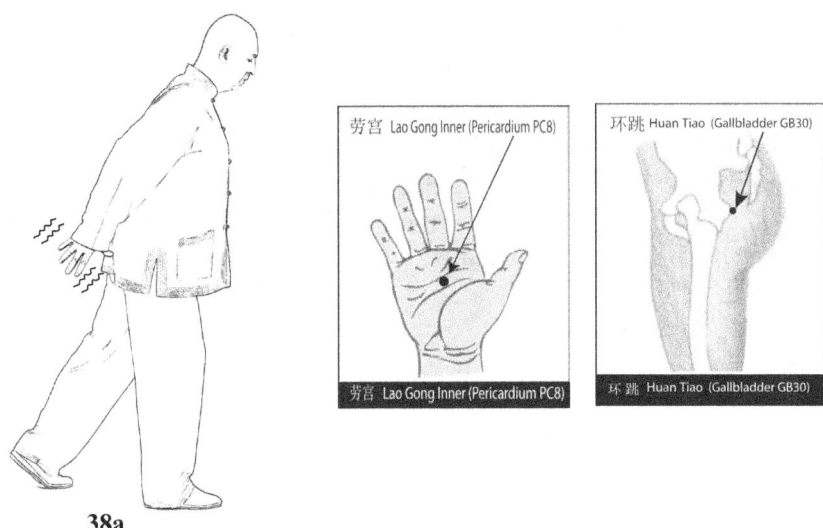

38a

38a　Move your bodyweight forward over the right leg, raising the left heel. Gently bend from the waist leaning the body at an angle of about 45°. At the same time, lower the fluttering arms down to the side of your body and open the chest sightly with arms rounded away from the body. Your arms are out wide behind the body with the Lao Gong (middle of palm) of both hands facing towards the Huan Tiao (indentation at side of hip).

Your eyes are looking down at a point about 2m in front of you. Stay in this position sensing the Qi for three seconds.

39. Swooping over the water 拍水飞翔

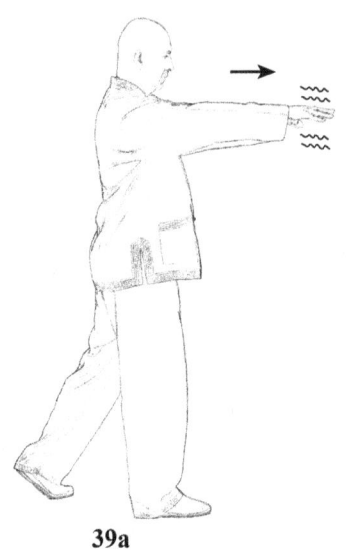

39a

39a   Slowly straighten your back by lifting the upper body. Raise the fluttering arms in front of your body to about shoulder height, facing toward the Southern direction. Relax your shoulders. Your arms are naturally rounded and the palms are turned in slightly. The Lao Gong (middle of palm) of both hands are facing each other.

Left swoop

39b   Move your bodyweight back over your left leg as the right heel comes off the ground. Turning from the waist gently swing both fluttering arms and swoop up to face the North East direction. The He Gu (web of hand) of both hands are facing each other and the hands are soft as if holding a small ball. Keep your shoulders and chest relaxed and look at the left hand which is in line with the head. The right hand is slightly lower and in line with the shoulder.

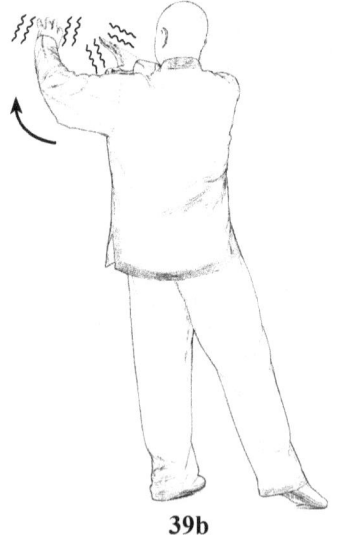

39b

Right swoop

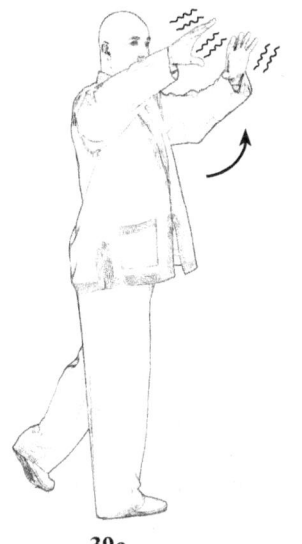

39c   Move your bodyweight forward over the right leg as the left heel comes off the ground. By turning at the waist, gently swing both fluttering arms down to about chest height and swoop up to face the South West direction. Both the He Gu (web of hand) are facing each other and the hands are soft as if holding a small ball. Keep your shoulders and chest relaxed and look at your right hand which is in line with the head. Your left hand is slightly lower and in line with the shoulder.

39c

Left swoop

39d   Move your bodyweight back over the left leg as the right heel comes off the ground. Turning from the waist, gently swing both fluttering arms down to about chest height and swoop up to face the North East direction. Both the He Gu (web of hand) are facing each other and the hands are soft as if holding a small ball. Keep your shoulders and chest relaxed and look at your left hand which is in line with the head. The right hand is slightly lower and in line with the shoulder.

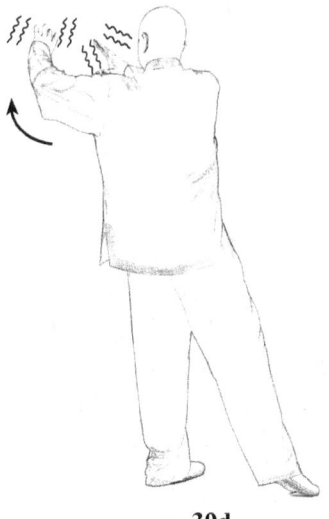

39d

40. Drinking the water 饮水

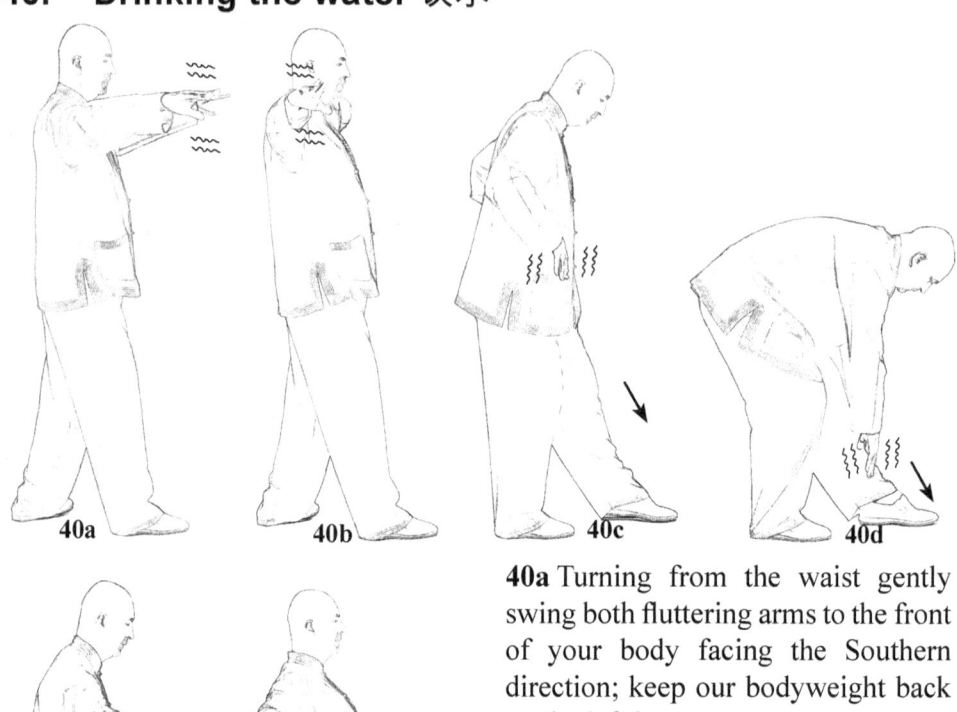

40a

40b

40c

40d

40e

40f

40a Turning from the waist gently swing both fluttering arms to the front of your body facing the Southern direction; keep our bodyweight back on the left leg.

40b,c Open fluttering arms to the side of your body and at the same time move your bodyweight over the right leg and step forward with the left toe just touching the ground.

40d Bend from the waist at an angle of about 45°, keeping all the weight on the right leg. The left leg is bent slightly with the toe just touching the ground. Move both fluttering arms down either side of the left leg down to the toes. The He Gu (web of hand) of both hands are facing each other creating an energy field down the leg. Your eyes are looking down following the hands as they move to the toes.

40e Slowly straighten your back by lifting the upper body. Your eyes are looking straight in front.

40f Raise fluttering arms to the side of your body to about waist height

Repeat three times.

Benefit: This movement benefits the throat, and is good for laryngitis and sinus problems. For throat problems breathe in and out through the mouth and for sinus problems breathe in and out through the nose.

41. Looking at the sky 望天

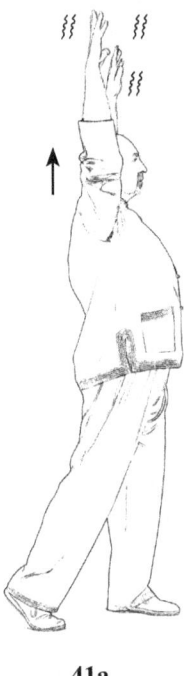

41a

41a　Gently move your bodyweight forward over the left leg as the right heel comes off the ground. At the same time, raise the fluttering wings up overhead. The palms are forward with the fingers to the sky. Keep your shoulders and elbows relaxed and arms about shoulder-width apart. Your eyes are looking up to the sky at an angle of about 45°. Stay in this position sensing the Qi for three seconds.

42. Recovering the Qi 归气

In this movement we are accumulating and refining the Qi and compressing it into the Lower Dan Tian (area beneath the navel) which helps stimulate the Qi through all parts of the body.

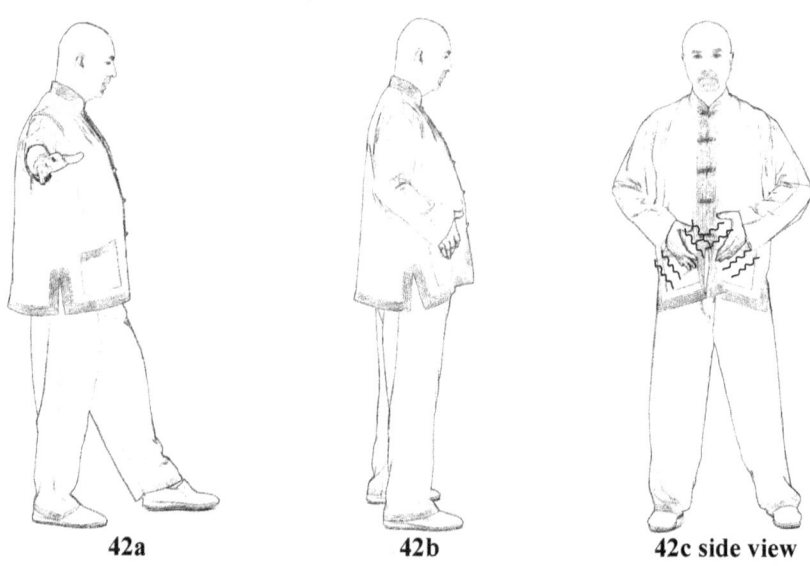

42a   42b   42c side view

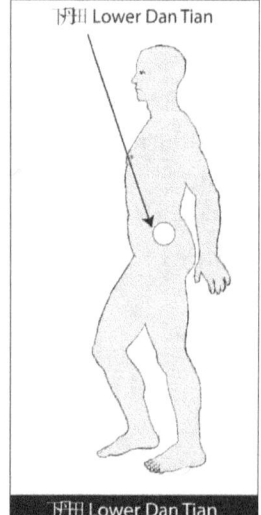

下丹田 Lower Dan Tian

下丹田 Lower Dan Tian

42a,b The right leg steps forward to be parallel with the left leg. The feet are about shoulder-width apart, weight evenly distributed. At the same time, lower both fluttering arms slowly to the side of your body, gradually reducing the quivering movement.

42c The palms turn in at the Lower Dan Tian (area beneath the navel). The hands are relaxed and hollow with the fingers gently separated and facing each other. The left hand is slightly higher than the right hand. Quiver the hands quickly three times and then sense the stillness for three seconds.

Repeat three times, sensing the stillness for three seconds in between each quiver.

43. Grasping the Qi 抓气

This movement receives and gathers Qi from nature and the external universe. If there is nothing natural within view from which to gather Qi, then visualise it. By bringing Qi to the chest area, the movement benefits the heart and lung.

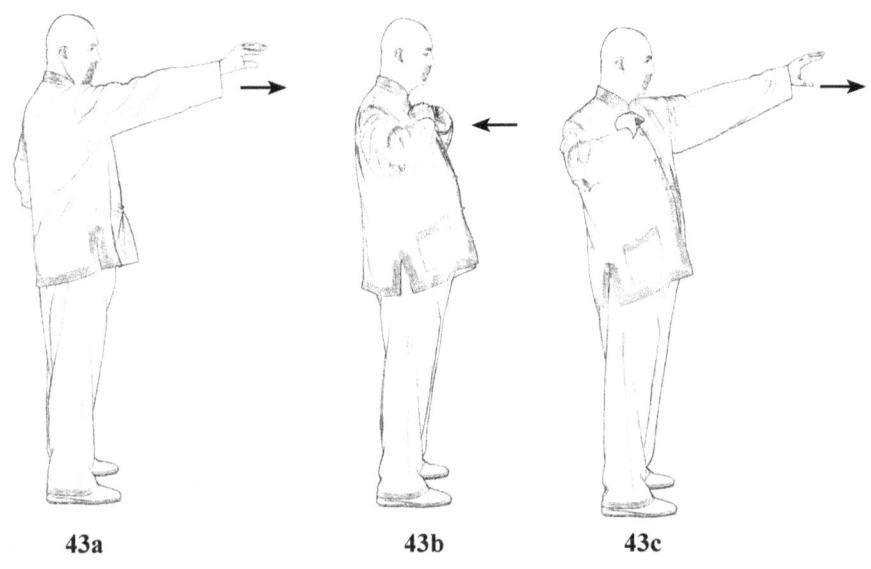

43a   **43b**   **43c**

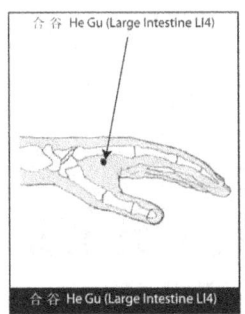

合谷 He Gu (Large Intestine LI4)

合谷 He Gu (Large Intestine LI4)

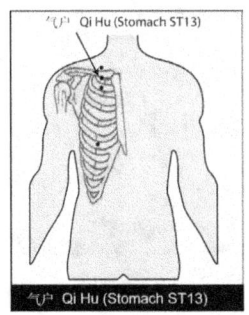

气户 Qi Hu (Stomach ST13)

气户 Qi Hu (Stomach ST13)

43a   Your feet remain about shoulder-width apart and your weight is evenly distributed. Your right arm reaches out in front to about shoulder height; your fingers are together, the thumb is relaxed and pointing down, and the palm is facing the earth. As the hand moves, your focus and awareness moves out to the distance. Keep your shoulders relaxed and your elbows off lock.

43b   Then gently clench the hand with the thumb and forefingers together forming a hollow fist and draw the elbow back. The He Gu (web of hand) gently touches the Qi Hu (beneath collar bone) as the mind focuses on the chest area.

43c   Repeat with the left hand for a total of ten movements – five to each side.

44.   Turning the palm up and grasping the Qi 翻掌搂气

In a similar way, this movement receives and gathers Qi from nature and the external universe. By bringing Qi to the chest area, the movement benefits the heart and lungs

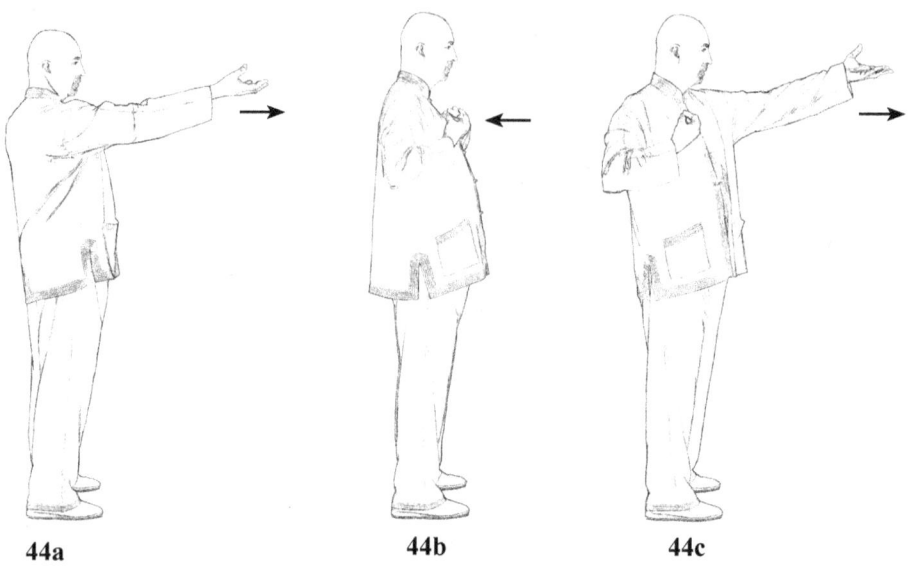

44a   **44b**   **44c**

44a   The right arm reaches out in front to about shoulder-height; your fingers are together, the thumb is relaxed and facing up, and the palm is facing the sky. As the hand moves, your focus and awareness moves out to the distance. Keep your shoulders relaxed and elbows off lock.

44b   Then gently clench the hand with the thumb and forefingers together forming a hollow fist, and draw the elbow back. The Hou Xi (Small Intestine SI3) on the outer edge of the palm in the middle of the hand gently touches the Ku Fang (Stomach ST14) between the collar bone and the nipple and one rib below the Qi Hu (beneath collar bone). Keep the mind focused on the chest area.

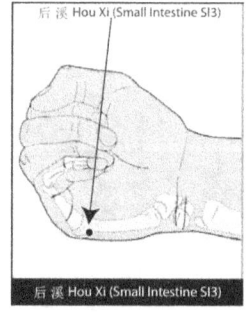

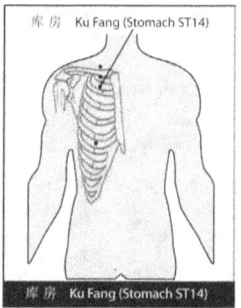

44c   Repeat the movement with the left hand.

Repeat for a total of ten movements – five to each side.

45.   Holding the Qi ball 抱球

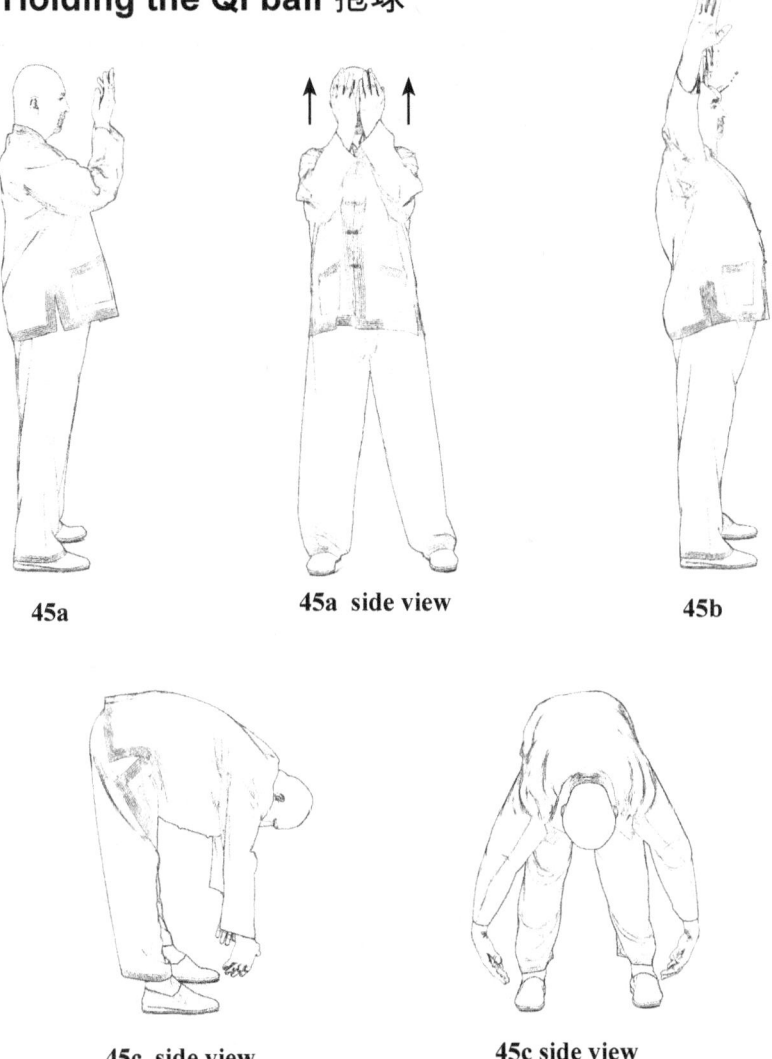

45a

45a side view

45b

45c side view

45c side view

45a,b Scoop the arms up in front of your body, with the palms turned towards your face.

45c   Keeping the legs straight, gently push the bottom back as you stretch forward and bend from the waist. Allow both arms to naturally hang in front of your body; elbows are rounded and the wrists are relaxed. The eyes are looking at the hands and the fingers are open and pointing to each other, as if holding a big ball in your arms. The Bai Hui at the top of the head is pointing forward.

46. Rotating the Qi ball 揉球

In movements 46 and 47, fresh Qi is received and stale Qi is dispersed. Rotating the Qi ball is like gently rolling the earth in your hands. It also stimulates the Qi around the Dai Mai Channel (waist area).

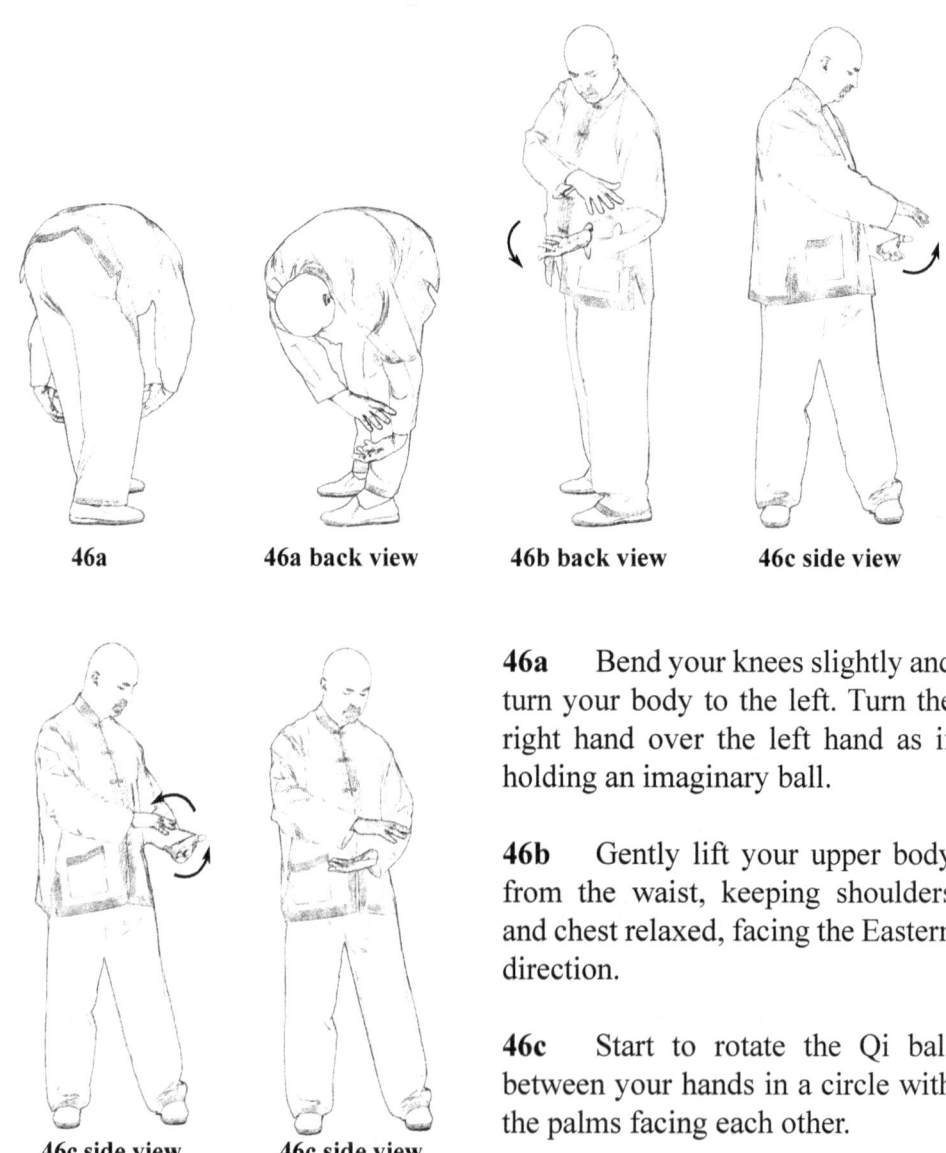

46a	**46a back view**	**46b back view**	**46c side view**

46c side view **46c side view**

46a Bend your knees slightly and turn your body to the left. Turn the right hand over the left hand as if holding an imaginary ball.

46b Gently lift your upper body from the waist, keeping shoulders and chest relaxed, facing the Eastern direction.

46c Start to rotate the Qi ball between your hands in a circle with the palms facing each other.

The bottom hand rotates out, allowing the stale Qi to go out and the top hand rotates in, allowing the fresh Qi to come in. The fingers are gently kneading the ball as your hands rotate, looking at the hands.

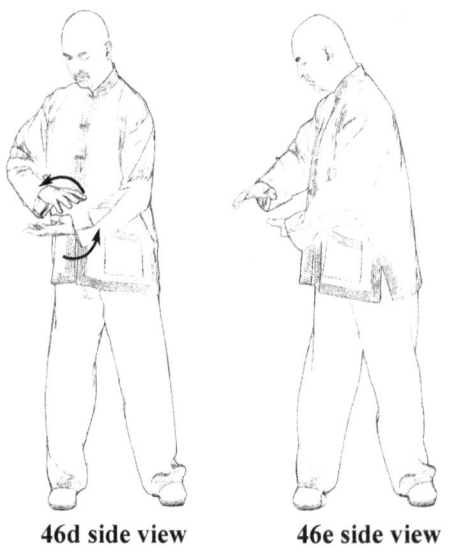

46d side view   46e side view

46d,e Turn your body slowly from the waist counting five rotations to face the Southern direction. Then continue turning, counting five more rotations to face the Western direction, looking at the hands all the time.

Benefit: The rotating movement benefits the pancreas, blood circulation and helps with insomnia. For people with insomnia this rotating hands movement can be done in private under the table whilst sitting down!

47. Turning the body and rotating the Qi ball 转身揉球

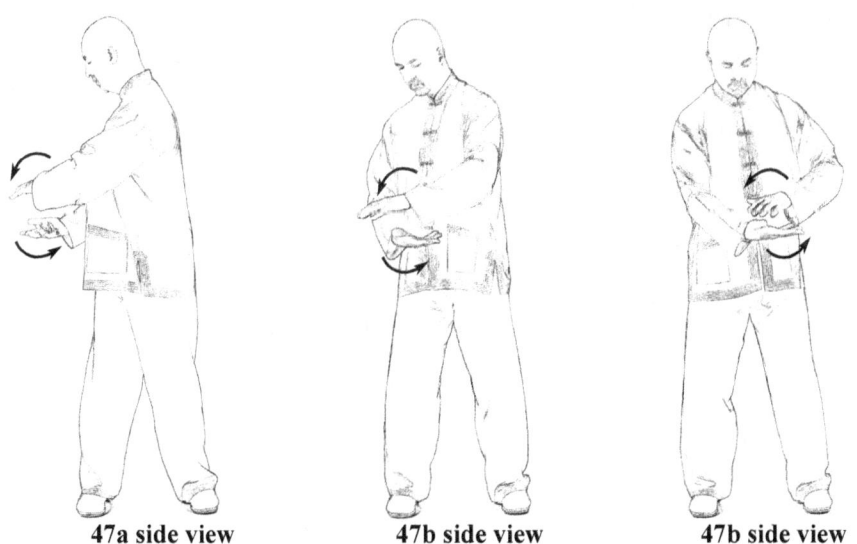

47a side view   47b side view   47b side view

47a Facing the Western direction, gently turn the hands over, being careful not to drop the Qi ball. The left hand is over the right hand while still holding the Qi ball. Start to rotate the Qi ball between the hands in a circle; the palms are facing each other. The bottom hand is rotating out, allowing the stale Qi to go out and the top hand is rotating in, allowing the fresh Qi to come in. The fingers are gently kneading the ball as the hands rotate; continue to look at the hands.

47b Turn your body slowly from the waist counting four rotations to face the Southern direction.

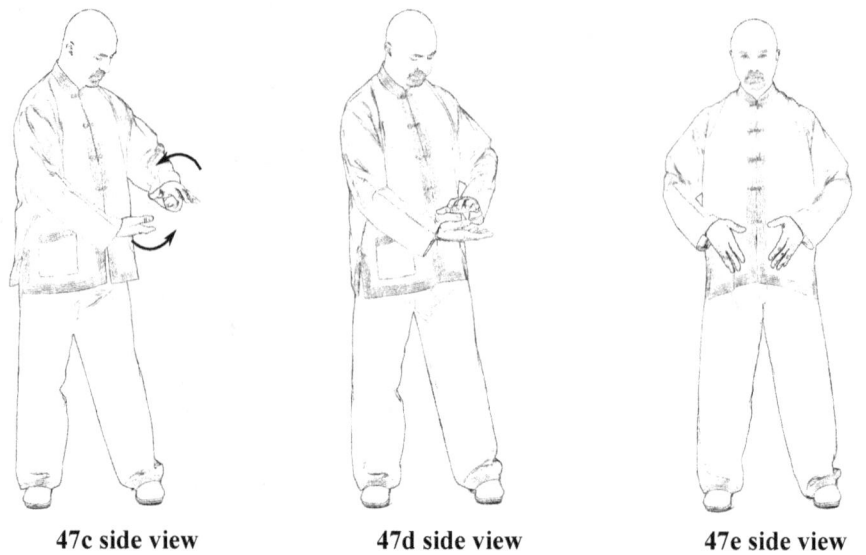

47c side view   **47d side view**   **47e side view**

47c   Continue turning your body counting four more rotations of the hands to face the Eastern direction, looking at the hands all the time.

47d   Keep the hands in the same position then count two more rotations to face the Southern direction.

47e   Relax your arms and turn the palms in to face the Lower Dan Tian (area beneath the navel). The arms and palms are at a distance of about 5cm from the body and your eyes are looking straight ahead.

48.   Holding the Qi 抱气

This is a strong movement that creates Yin/Yang balance. Qi is lifted from the earth to nurture the whole energy system of the body. It helps to regulate all the organs.

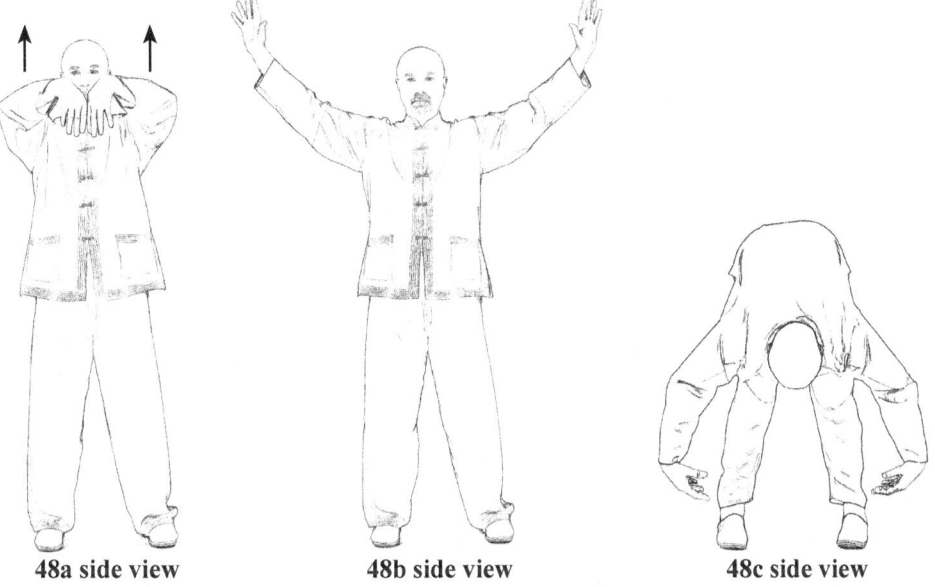

| 48a side view | 48b side view | 48c side view |

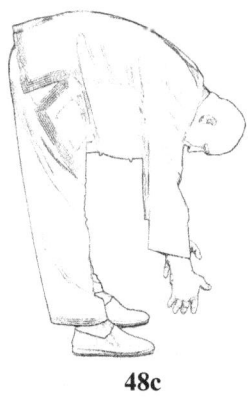

48c

48a   Raise the arms in front of your body, with the palms turned towards the face and fingers pointing to the ground. The He Gu (web of hand) of both hands are facing each other.

48b Keeping your shoulders and elbows relaxed, separate the arms and swing both palms out in a circle to the side of the body.

48c Straighten your legs and gently push the bottom back as you stretch forward and bend from the waist. Allow both arms to naturally hang in front of the body; elbows are rounded and the wrists relaxed. Your eyes are looking at the hands and the fingers are open and pointing to each other, as if holding a big heavy ball in your arms. The Bai Hui (top of the head) is pointing forward. In this movement we are lifting Yin Qi from the earth to make a Qi field to nurture five organs – Heart, Lung, Liver, Kidney and Spleen.

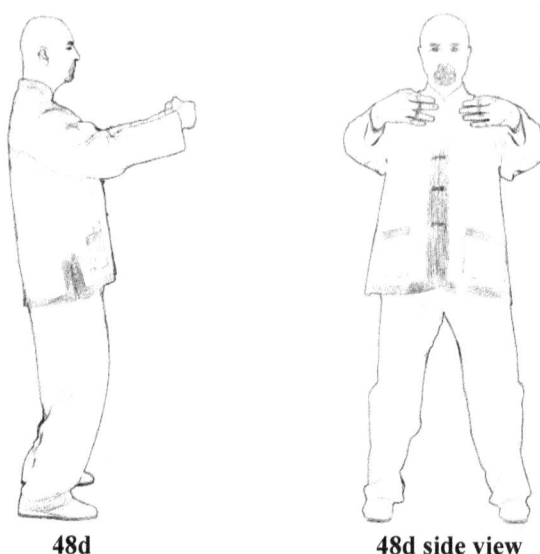

48d   48d side view

48d   Gently bend your knees and lift your upper body from the waist, keeping your shoulders and chest relaxed. Your bodyweight is evenly distributed as the knees lower to the ground; the arms are still holding a large heavy ball. This movement nurtures Yin and Yang. The Lao Gong (middle of palm) face towards the Qi Hu (beneath collar bone). Stay in this position for three seconds. Your eyes are looking straight ahead.

49. Distributing the Qi 贯气

These movements distribute Qi from the head down through the whole body.

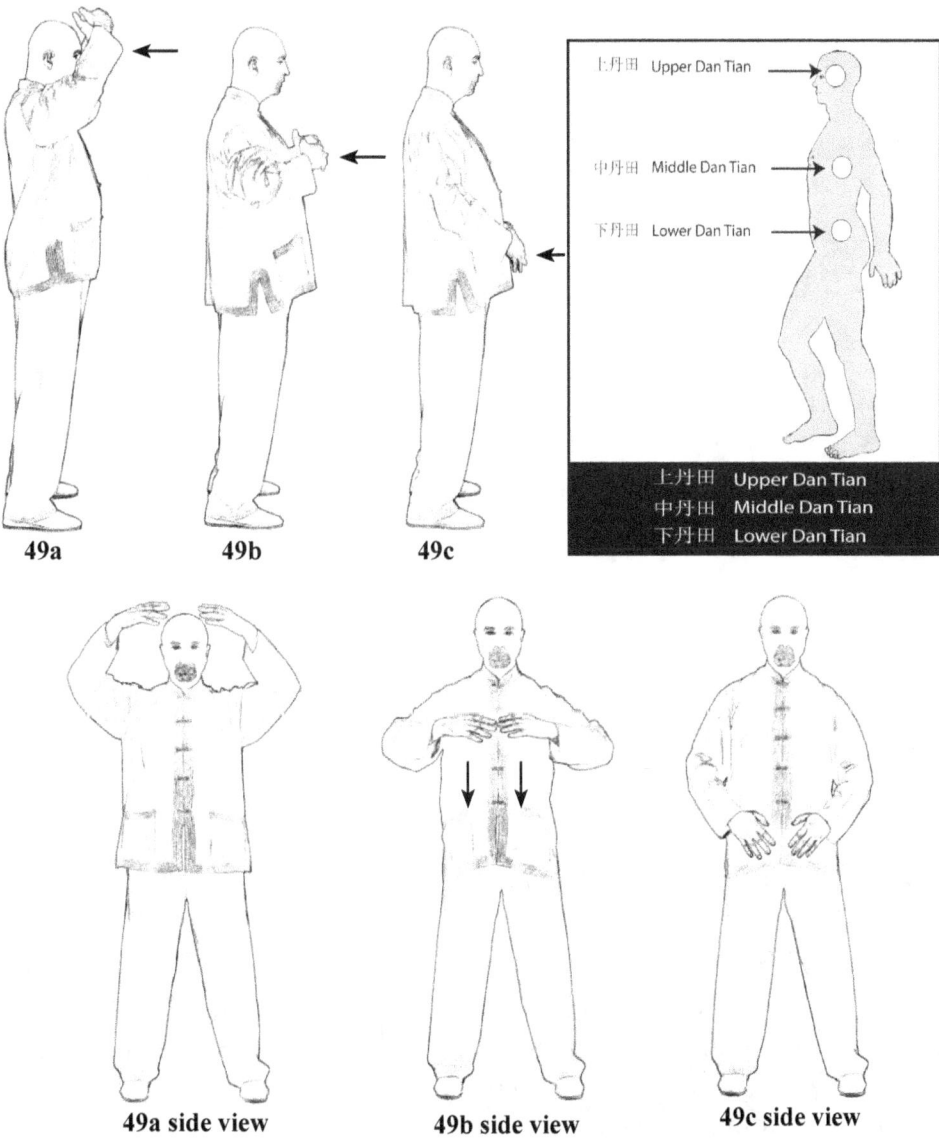

上丹田	Upper Dan Tian
中丹田	Middle Dan Tian
下丹田	Lower Dan Tian

49a   49b   49c

49a side view   49b side view   49c side view

49a,b,c Raise your body slightly by gently straightening the legs. Your arms rise up with the body still hol ding the ball of Qi towards the forehead. Your arms slowly descend in front of your body as the palms regulate and distribute the Qi into the Upper Dan Tian (between the eyebrows) pause for a few seconds, the Middle Dan Tian (middle of chest between the nipples) pause for a few seconds, and the Lower Dan Tian (area beneath the navel), pause for a few seconds.

50.   Thrusting out the wings 抬膀

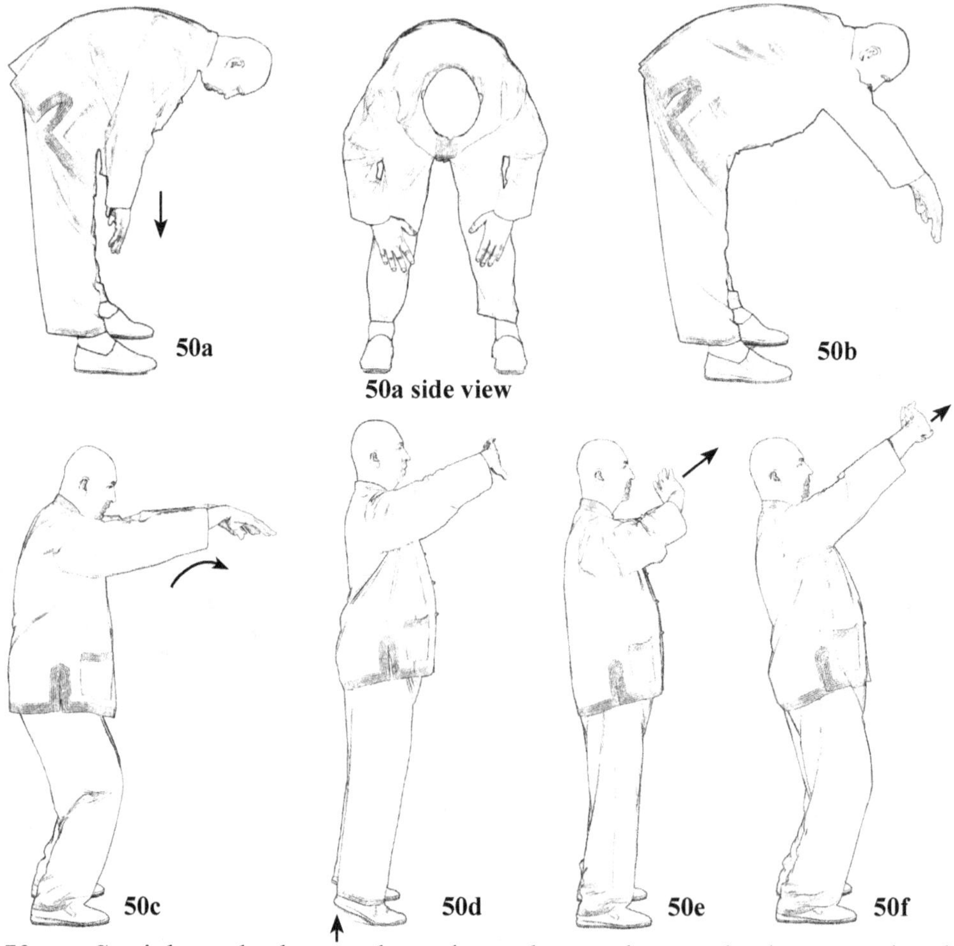

50a

50a side view

50b

50c   50d   50e   50f

50a   Straighten the legs and gently push your bottom back as you bend from the waist and stretch forward. The hands slowly scan down the inside of both legs to the feet.

50b,c,d Gently bend your knees and lift your upper body from the waist, keeping your shoulders and chest relaxed. The arms rise up over your head in coordination with the body. Your bodyweight moves forward onto the balls of both feet, lifting the heels.

50e   Quickly thrust your arms forward with the palms facing outward at about the height of your forehead. The shoulders and chest are relaxed and arms slightly rounded with the He Gu (web of hand) of both hands facing each other to maintain the energy field. At the same time, move your bodyweight back, making a sharp, stomping and forceful movement, grounding your bodyweight onto both heels.

Benefit: Movements 45 to 50 are good for the head and chest.

51. Turning over the wings 翻翅

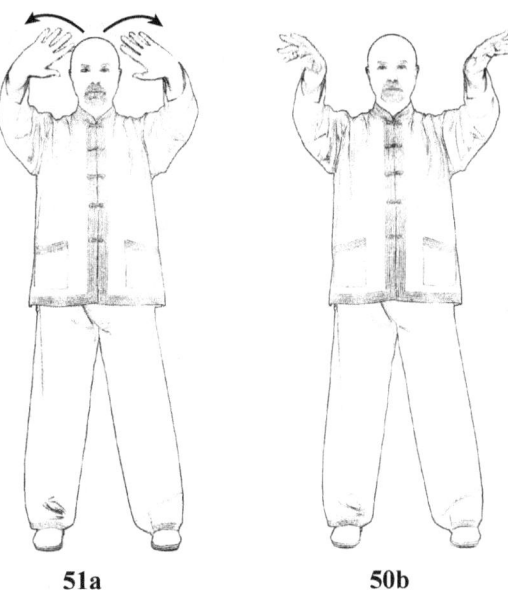

51a   50b

51a,b Relax both hands and turn both wrists outward in a circle forming the Plum Blossom Claw (four fingers touching together with the thumb) with both hands. Drop the elbows and bring them closer to the body to draw the Qi into the Plum Blossom Claw.

52. Bringing the wings to the back 背翅

This balances Yin and Yang energy and enables the Qi to drop down to the Yong Quan (Kidney K1) at the soles of the feet.

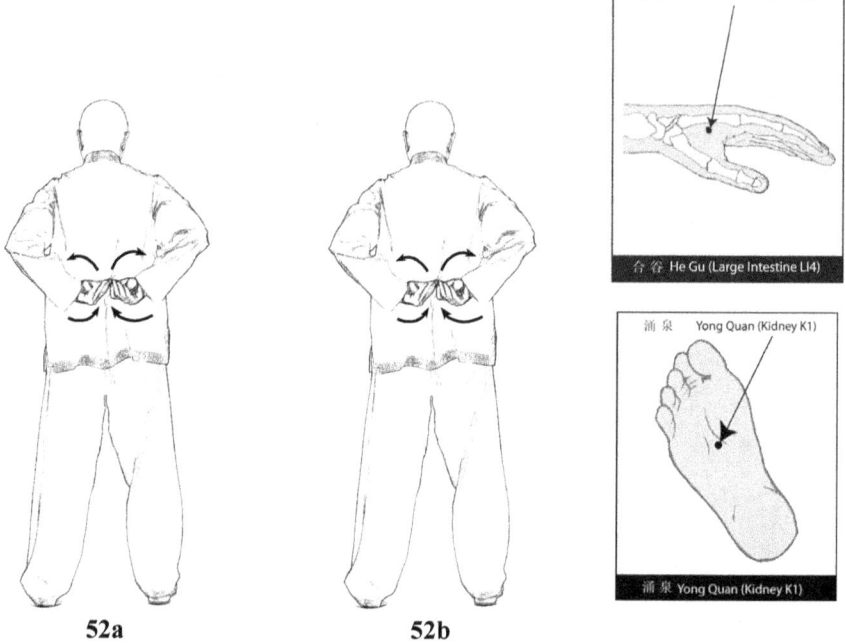

52a   **52b**

52a   Circle both arms backward and behind your body. Relax the elbows and gently touch the He Gu (web of hand) to the Shen Shu (beneath the Kidneys).

52b   Relax the hands as the He Gu (web of hand) gently massages the Shen Shu (beneath the Kidneys) rotating three times and then pausing for three seconds.

Repeat the set of three rotations three times, pausing between each massage.

53. Flying up to the side 起扇上飞

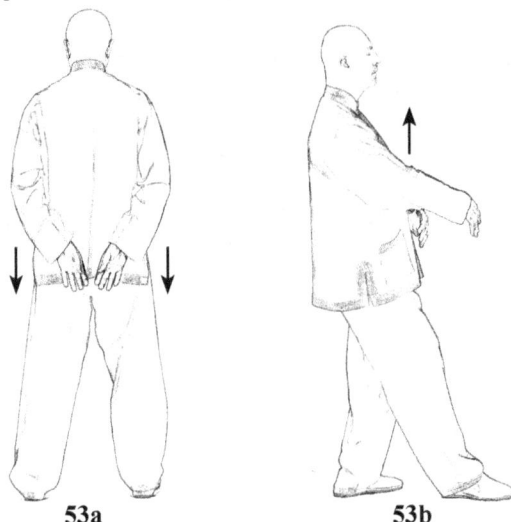

53a   53b

53a   Relaxing both arms allow the hands to move down the back of the body. Circle both arms forward and around in front of the body.

53b   Your shoulders are relaxed and the elbow is at an angle of about 90°. The fingers are open and the hands are naturally relaxed. The left hand is closer to the body than the right hand which is on the outside at a distance of about 3cm from the left hand. Cross the hands at the palms with the Lao Gong (middle of palm) of both hands connecting.

Repeat the left and right movements for a total of seven times.

Benefit: These 'flying up to the side' movements exercise the wrists and shoulders and improve the function of blood vessels through the whole body. They also benefit the Liver and Gall Bladder.

Movements 53 to 58 are good for the head and chest.

Flying up to the left

In all these movements, the Lao Gong (palm of hand) is facing the body and drawing Qi up the Ren Channel (front line of the body).

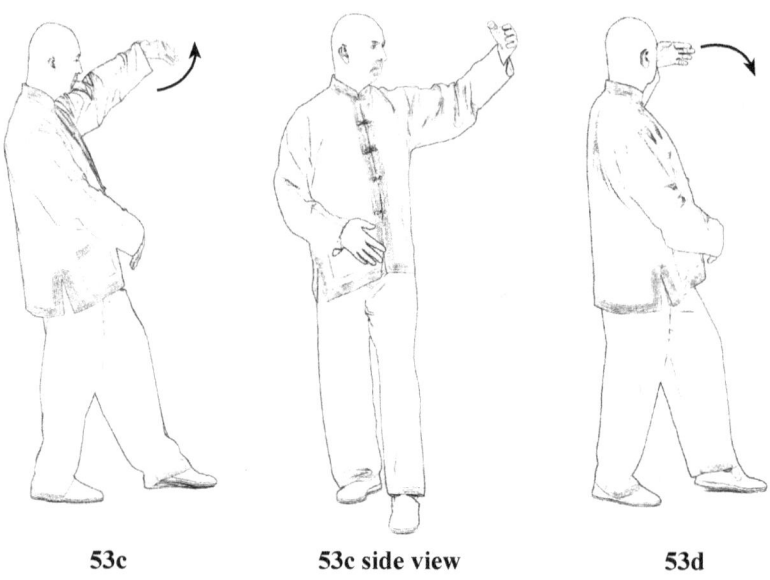

53c   53c side view   53d

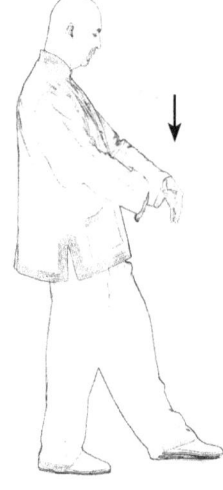

53c   Move your bodyweight to the right leg and gently step forward with the left foot, the outer edge of the foot (small toe) just touching. At the same time, raise your left arm keeping the shoulder and elbow relaxed to the height of the forehead.

53d   Moving from the waist, turn your body to the Eastern direction with your eyes following the hand; feel the warmth in the back of the neck.

53e   Turn your body from the waist back to the front, facing the Southern direction. The left arm circles down in front of the abdomen on the outside of the right arm. Cross the hands at the palms at a distance of about 3cm, connecting the Lao Gong (middle of palm).

53e

Flying up to the right

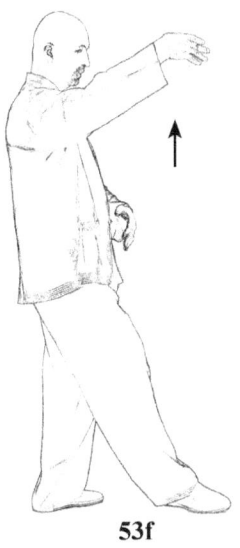

53f

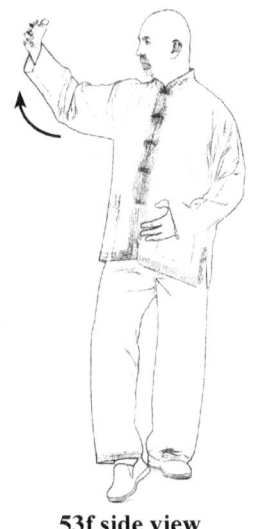

53f side view

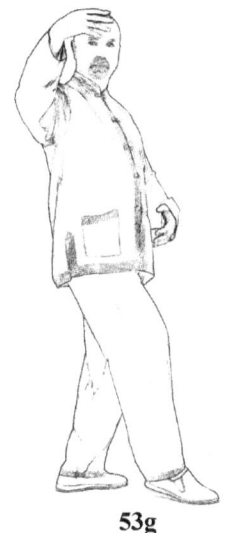

53g

53f Move your bodyweight to the left foot and gently step forward with the right foot, the outer edge of the foot (small toe) just touching. At the same time, raise your right arm keeping the shoulder and elbow relaxed to the height of the forehead.

53g Moving from the waist, turn your body to the Western direction with your eyes following the hand; feel the warmth in the back of the neck.

53h Turn your body from the waist back to the front, facing the Southern direction. The right arm circles down in front of the abdomen on the outside of the left arm. Cross the hands at the palms at a distance of about 3cm, connecting the Lao Gong (middle of palm).

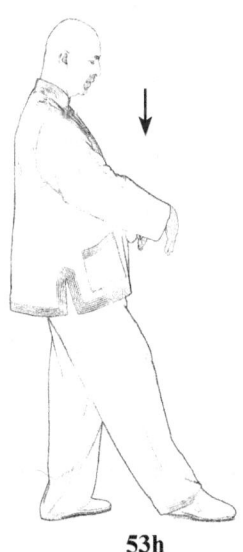

53h

Flying up to the left

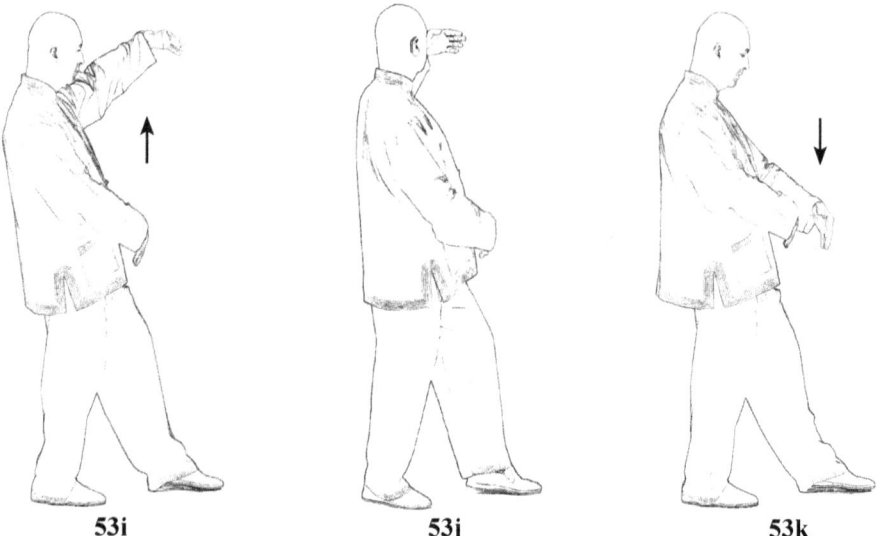

53i   53j   53k

53i   Move your bodyweight to the right leg and gently step forward with the left foot, the outer edge of the foot (small toe) just touching. At the same time, raise your left arm keeping the shoulder and elbow relaxed to the height of the forehead.

53j   Moving from the waist, turn your body to the Eastern direction with your eyes following the hand; feel the warmth in the back of the neck.

53k   Turn your body from the waist back to the front, facing the Southern direction. The left arm circles down in front of the abdomen on the outside of the right arm. Cross the hands at the palms at a distance of about 3cm, connecting the Lao Gong (middle of palm).

Repeat the left and right movements for a total of seven times.

54. Turning the body 转身

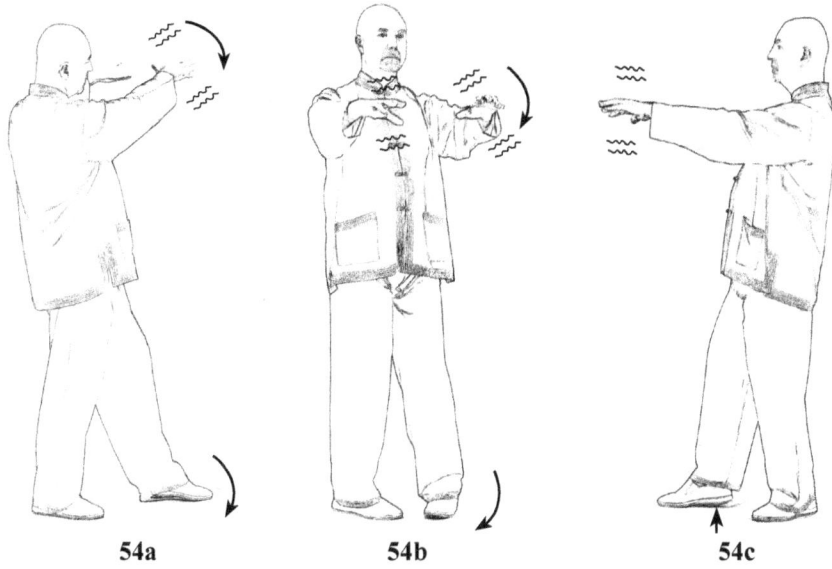

54a   54b   54c

54a   Your bodyweight remains on the right leg after the seventh Fly up to the side movement. Turn your body from the waist to the South East direction and raise both fluttering arms to about shoulder height. Keep your shoulders and chest relaxed with the He Gu (web of hand) of both hands facing each other. The hands are no wider than shoulder-width apart.

54b   Turn your body 180° to face the Northern direction. Pivoting on your left heel, hook the left toe in as far as feels comfortable. Slightly bend your left knee and move your bodyweight back over the left leg, pivoting on your right toe.

54c   Your right toe is just touching the ground and both fluttering arms are in front of your body at shoulder height. Your eyes are looking straight ahead.

55. Flying up 飞上

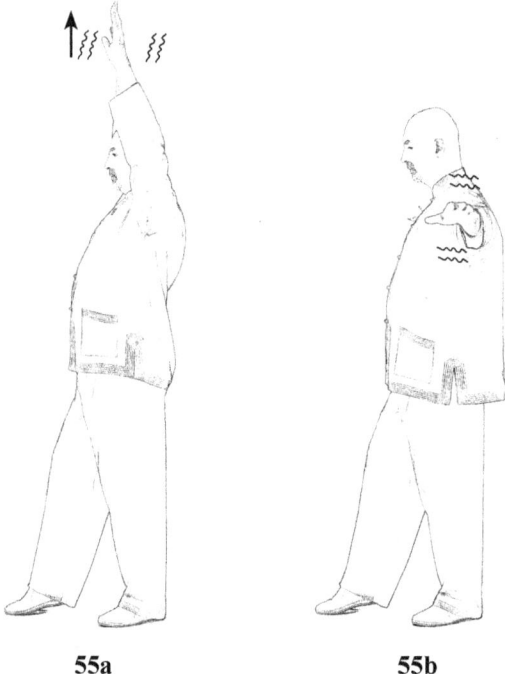

55a   55b

55a   Raise both fluttering arms up over your head, keeping shoulders and elbows relaxed. Your palms are facing forward and fingers are pointing toward the sky. The arms are slightly rounded with the He Gu (web of hand) of both hands facing each other. The hands are no wider than shoulder-width apart. Stay in this position for three seconds with your eyes looking straight ahead.

55b   Slowly lower your fluttering arms to the side of your body at about shoulder height, keeping shoulders and elbows relaxed.

56. Flying over the water 过水飞翔

These movements turn and twist from the waist swinging the upper body to face and absorb the Qi from the eight directions of the Bagua.

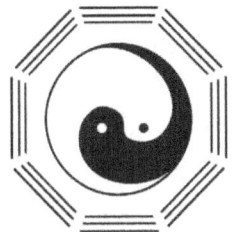

Bagua: The Bagua represents the eight directions of the compass: North, North East, East, South East, South, South West, West, North West.

Flying to the left

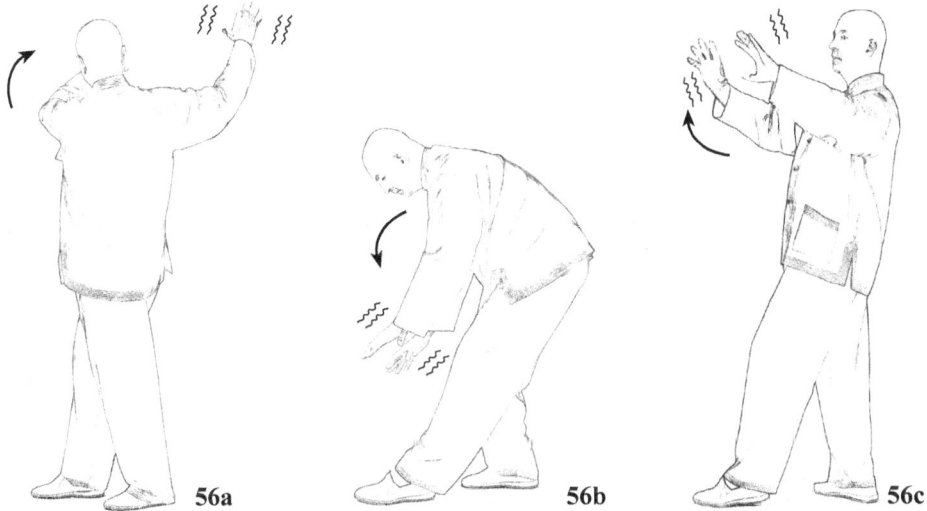

56a   56b   56c

56a Keeping your bodyweight on the left leg gently swing both fluttering arms turning from the waist and fly up to face the South East direction. The He Gu (web of hand) of both hands are facing each other. Keeping your shoulders and chest relaxed, look at the right hand which is in line with your head; the left hand is slightly lower in line with the shoulder.

56b Move your bodyweight over the right leg and gently swing both fluttering arms to the left, turning from the waist and crouching forward at an angle of about 45°.

56c Keeping your bodyweight over the right leg the quivering hands pass below the knee and fly up to face the North West direction. Both the He Gu (web of hand) are facing each other. Keeping shoulders and chest relaxed, look at your left hand which is in line with your head and your right hand is slightly lower in line with your shoulder.

Flying to the right

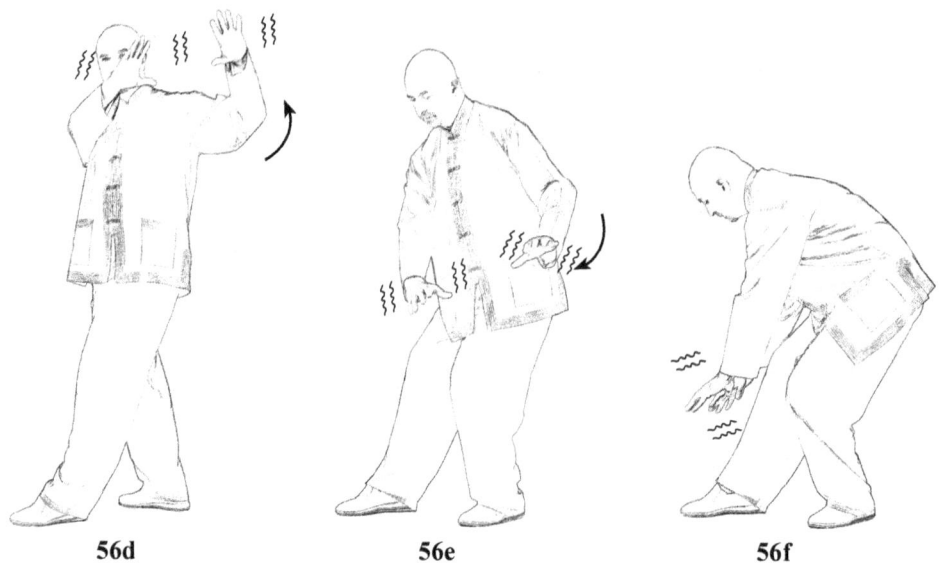

56d   56e   56f

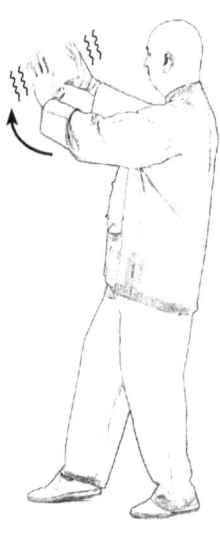

56g

56d   Maintaining your bodyweight on the right leg, turn from the waist and gently swing both fluttering arms to the left facing the South West direction.

56e   Move your bodyweight to the left leg and gently step forward with the right foot, toe just touching the ground.

56f   Gently swing both fluttering arms to the right, turning from the waist and crouching forward at an angle of about 45°.

56g   Keeping your bodyweight over the left leg the quivering hands pass below the knee and fly up to face the North East direction. The He Gu (web of hand) of both hands are facing each other. Keeping your shoulders and chest relaxed, look at your right hand which is in line with your head; your left hand is slightly lower in line with your shoulder.

Flying to the left

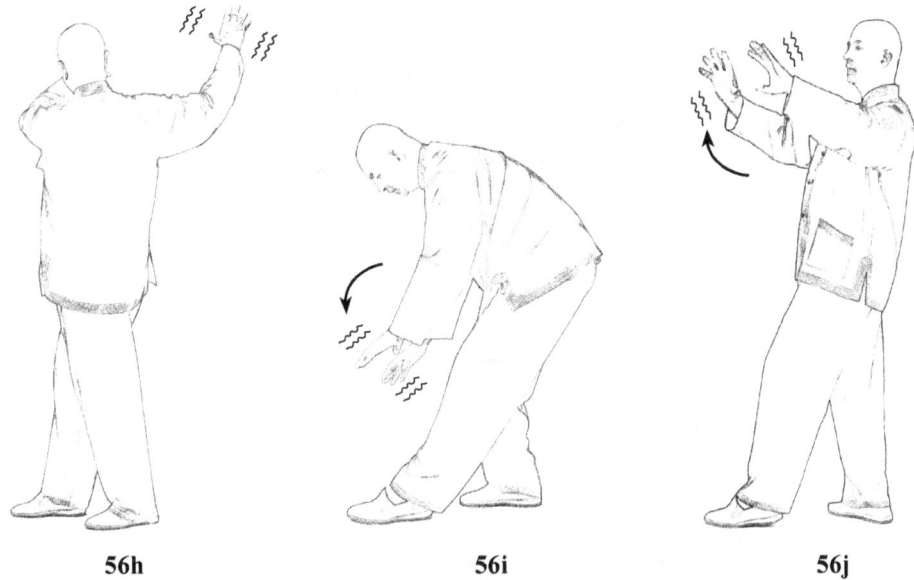

56h   **56i**   **56j**

56h   Keeping your bodyweight on the left leg gently swing both fluttering arms turning from the waist and fly up to face the South East direction. The He Gu (web of hand) of both hands are facing each other. Keeping your shoulders and chest relaxed, look at the right hand which is in line with your head; the left hand is slightly lower in line with the shoulder.

56i   Move your bodyweight over the right leg and gently swing both fluttering arms to the left, turning from the waist and crouching forward at an angle of about 45°.

56j   Keeping your bodyweight over the right leg the quivering hands pass below the knee and fly up to face the North West direction. Both the He Gu (web of hand) are facing each other. Keeping shoulders and chest relaxed, look at your left hand which is in line with your head and your right hand is slightly lower in line with your shoulder.

Repeat for a total of seven times; finish facing the North West direction.

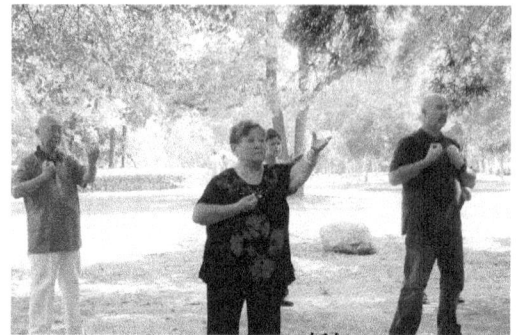

Grasping the Qi 抓气

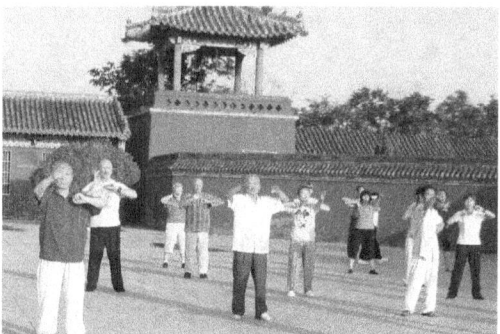

Turning palm up and grasping the Qi　落榜回气

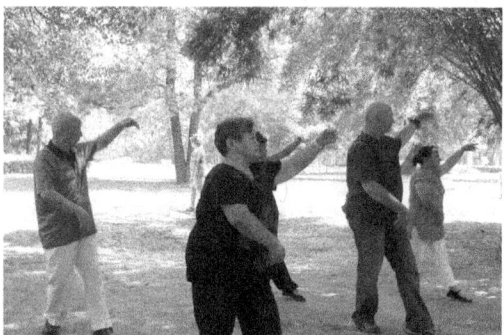

Flying up to the side　　起扇上飞

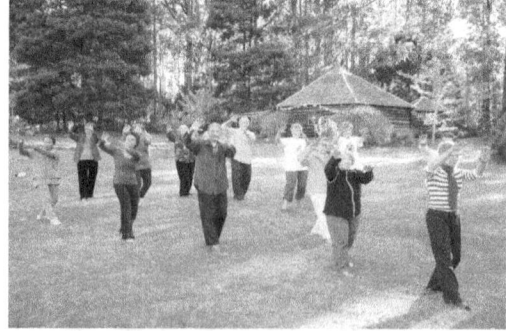

Flying over the water　过水飞翔

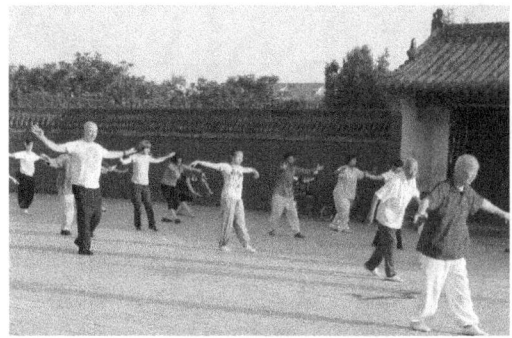

Looking for the food 寻食

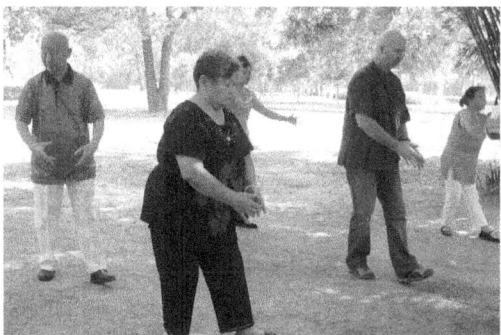

Turning the body 转身

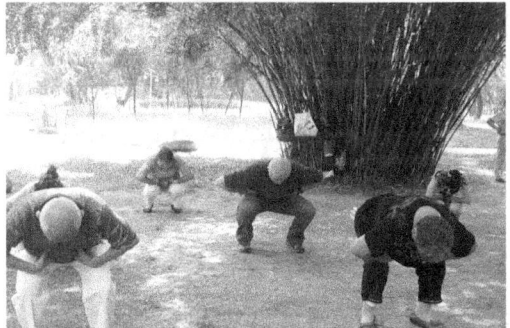

Sleeping peacefully and recovering the Qi 安睡归气

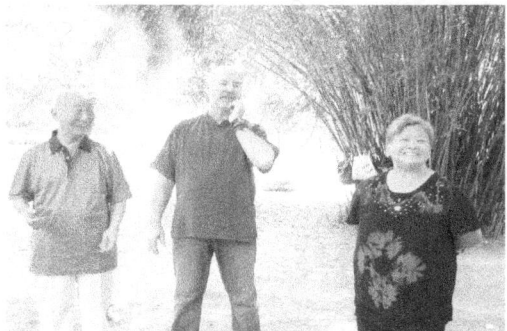

Master, Madam Chen and Simon Blow

57. Turning the body 转身

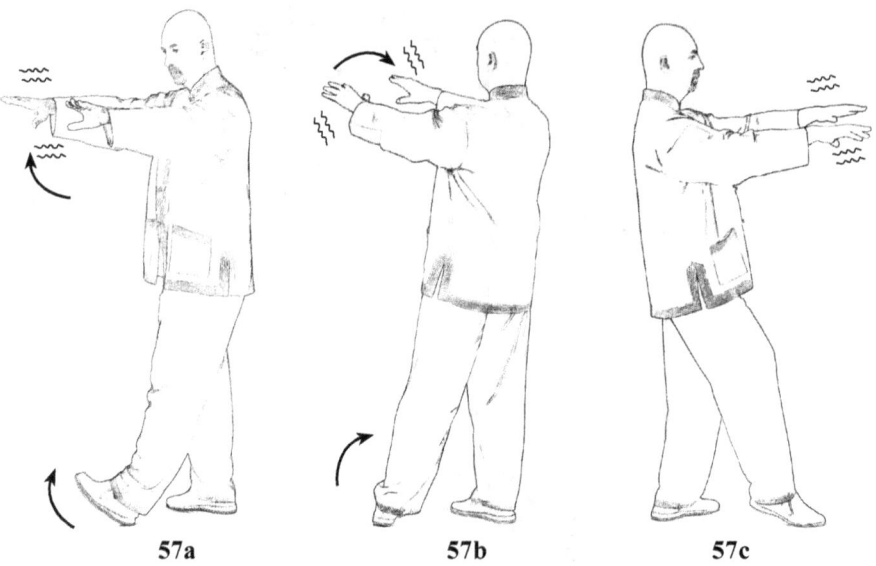

57a   57b   57c

57a   Your bodyweight remains on the right leg after the seventh Fly over the water movement.

57b   Turn your body 180° to face the Southern direction. Pivoting on your left heel, hook the left toe in as far as feels comfortable. Slightly bend the left knee and move your bodyweight back over the left leg, pivoting on the right toe.

57c   The right toe is just touching the ground and both fluttering arms are in front of your body at shoulder height; the eyes are looking straight ahead.

58. Flying up 飞上

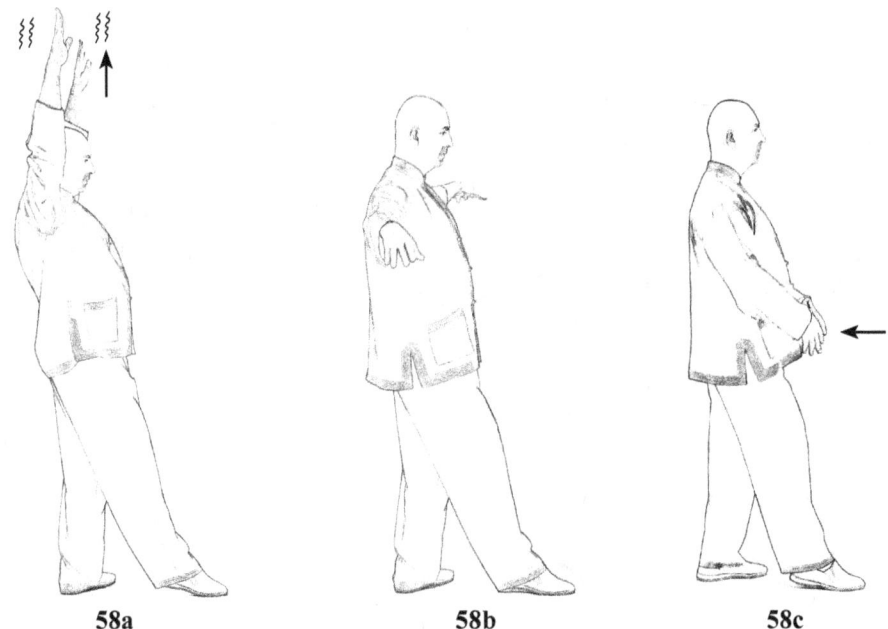

58a   58b   58c

58a   Raise both fluttering arms up over your head, keeping the shoulders and elbows relaxed. Your palms are facing forward and the fingers are pointing toward the sky. The He Gu of both hands (web of hand) are facing each other. The hands are no wider than shoulder-width apart. Stay in this position for three seconds with the eyes looking straight ahead.

58b   Slowly lower your arms to the side of your body at about shoulder height and reduce the fluttering to a complete stop. Keep shoulders, elbows and wrists relaxed with the fingers pointing naturally to the ground.

58c   Lower your arms with the palms facing the Lower Dan Tian (area beneath the navel).

59.   Looking for the food 寻食

According to Master Chen, this is one of the most powerful movements of the 1st 64 movement set. By gathering the heaven Qi and connecting to the earth Qi these movements strengthen the Lower Dan Tian (area beneath the navel) and stimulate the Small and Large Orbit.

Benefit: These movements have many healing benefits including strengthening spine health, reducing cardiovascular disease, stimulating the Kidneys and the Large Intestine, aiding fertility and boosting the immune system.

Looking for food to the left

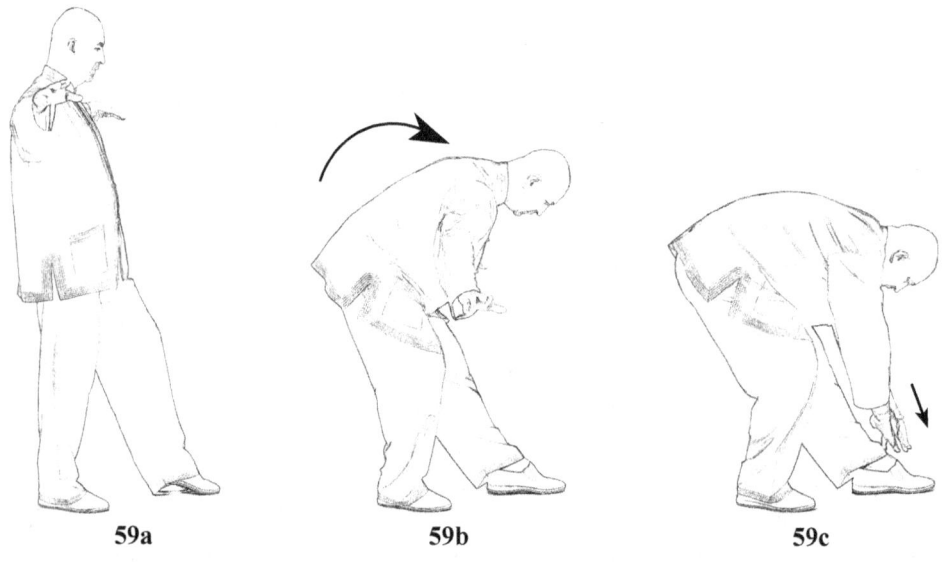

59a   59b   59c

59a   Facing the Southern direction, move your bodyweight to the right leg and gently step forward with the left foot, toe just touching the ground. At the same time, gently lift both arms (wings) to the side.

59b,c Bend from the waist, crouching forward at an angle of about 45°. Your arms swing down over your left foot. The left hand is on top of the right hand with the fingers pointing straight ahead. The distance between the hands is about 3cm and the right hand is about 3cm above the foot. Connect the Lao Gong (middle of palm) of each hand.

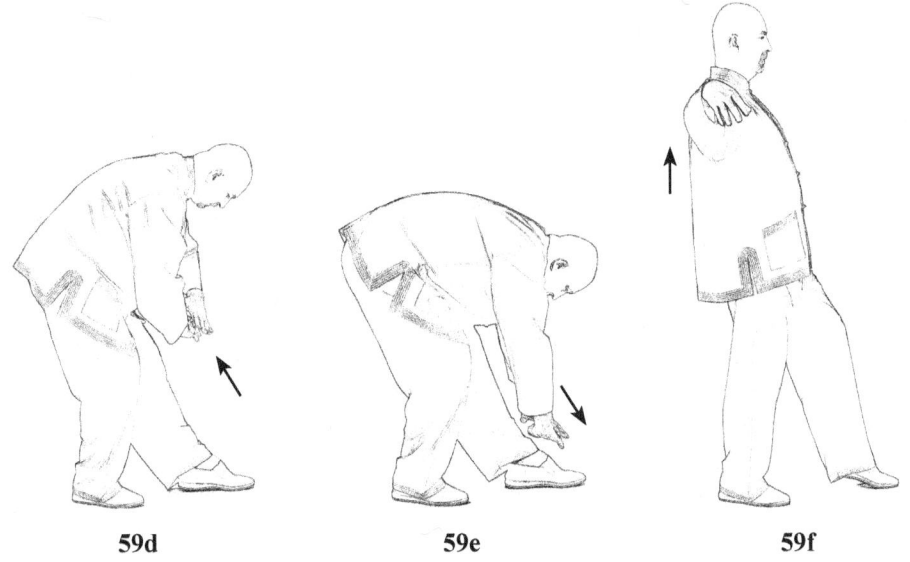

| 59d | 59e | 59f |

59d   Lift the upper body slightly from the waist, drawing the crossed hands up to the knee while gently bending the elbows.

59e   Pushing down from the waist, the crossed hands push down over your left foot.

59f   Lift the upper body from the waist, and at the same time gently lift both arms (wings) to the side. Your eyes are looking straight ahead.

Looking for food to the right

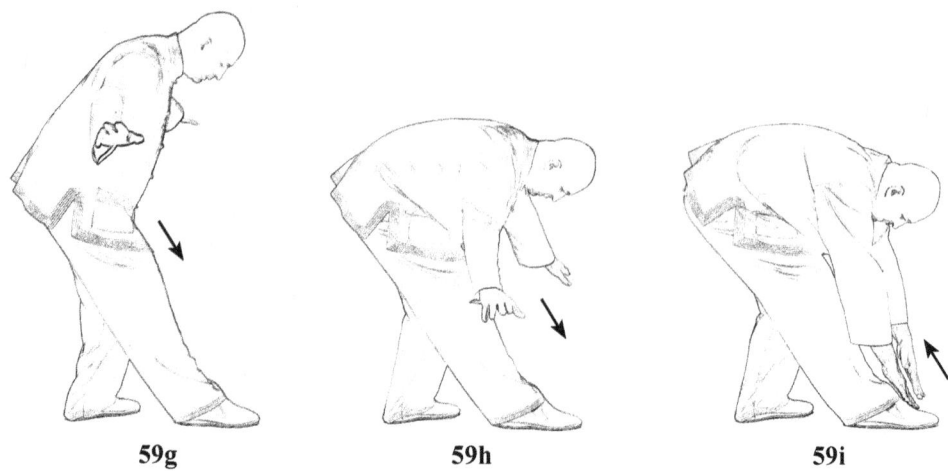

59g   59h   59i

59g   Move your bodyweight to the left leg and gently step forward with the right foot, toe just touching the ground.

59h,i   Bend from the waist, crouching forward at an angle of about 45°. Your arms swing down over your right foot. The left hand is on top of the right hand with the fingers pointing straight ahead. The distance between the hands is about 3cm and the right hand is about 3cm above the foot. Connect the Lao Gong (middle of palm) of each hand.

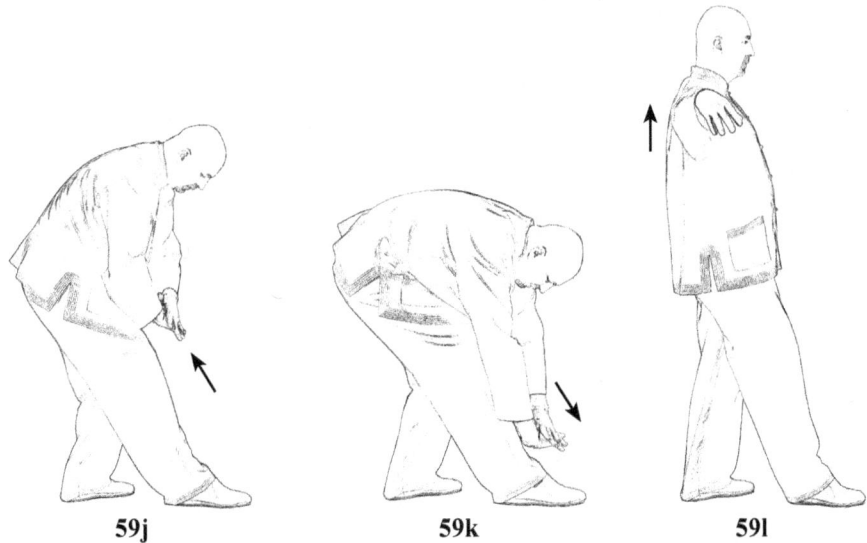

59j　　Lift the upper body slightly from the waist, drawing the crossed hands up to the knee while gently bending the elbows.

59k　　Pushing down from the waist, the crossed hands push down over your right foot.

59l　　Lift the upper body from the waist, and at the same time gently lift both arms (wings) to the side. Your eyes are looking straight ahead.

Looking for food to the left

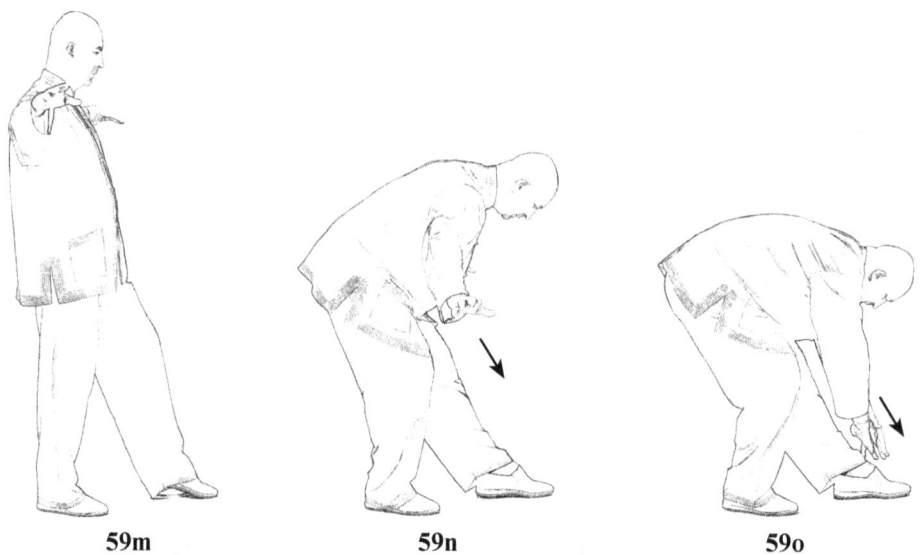

59m 59n 59o

59m   Facing the Southern direction, move your bodyweight to the right leg and gently step forward with the left foot, toe just touching the ground. At the same time, gently lift both arms (wings) to the side.

59n,o   Bend from the waist, crouching forward at an angle of about 45°. Your arms swing down over your left foot. The left hand is on top of the right hand with the fingers pointing straight ahead. The distance between the hands is about 3cm and the right hand is about 3cm above the foot. Connect the Lao Gong (middle of palm) of each hand.

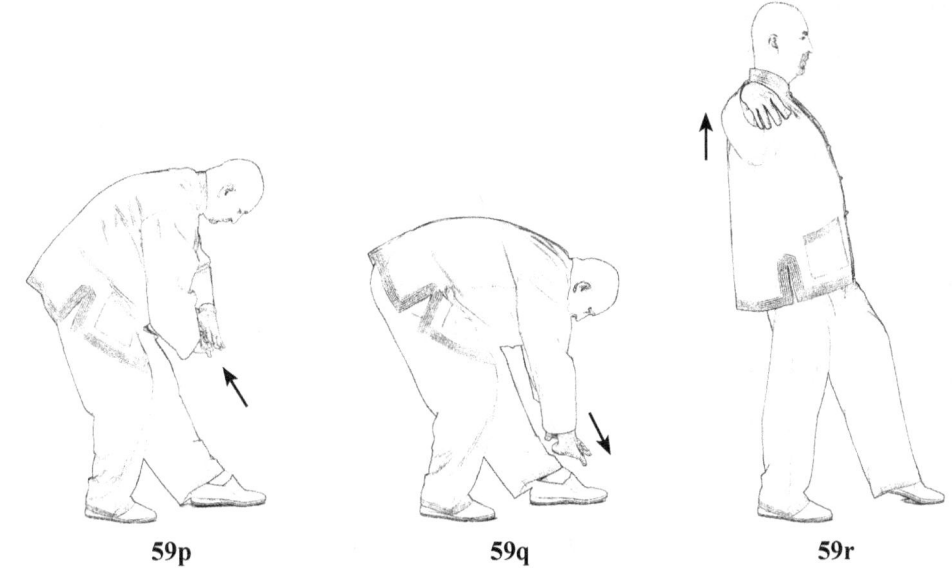

59p   Lift the upper body slightly from the waist, drawing the crossed hands up to the knee while gently bending the elbows.

59q   Pushing down from the waist, the crossed hands push down over your left foot.

59r   Lift the upper body from the waist, and at the same time gently lift both arms (wings) to the side. Your eyes are looking straight ahead.

Repeat for a total of seven times.

60.   Turning the body 转身

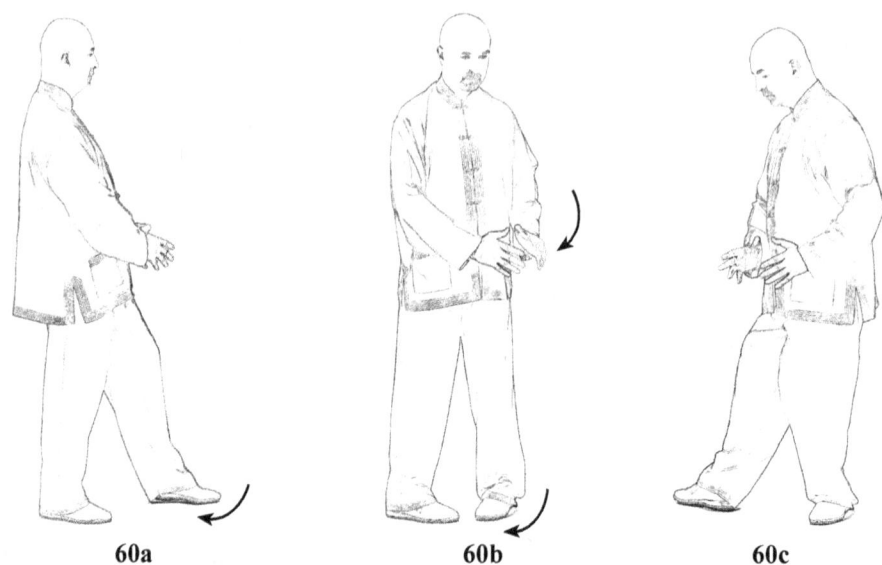

60a   **60b**   **60c**

60a   Your bodyweight remains on the right leg after the seventh 'Looking for the food' movement.

60b   Turn your body 180° to face the Northern direction. Pivoting on the left heel, hook in your left toe as far as feels comfortable. Bend your knees slightly so you don't twist and hurt the knees. The left toes are facing the North West direction.

60c   Move your bodyweight back onto the left leg and pivot on the right heel turning the right toe to face the North East direction.

At the same time, the arms raise up with the body, keeping shoulders, chest and elbows relaxed. Your palms are facing each other holding a Qi ball or 'egg' in the hands, in front of the Lower Dan Tian (area beneath the navel).

61. Looking for the nest 寻窝

This is an important movement in preparation for processing the Qi before the closing movement. Each movement is done slowly and deliberately, drawing Qi from the earth and allowing it to be absorbed by the body and refined.

No. 1 to the left

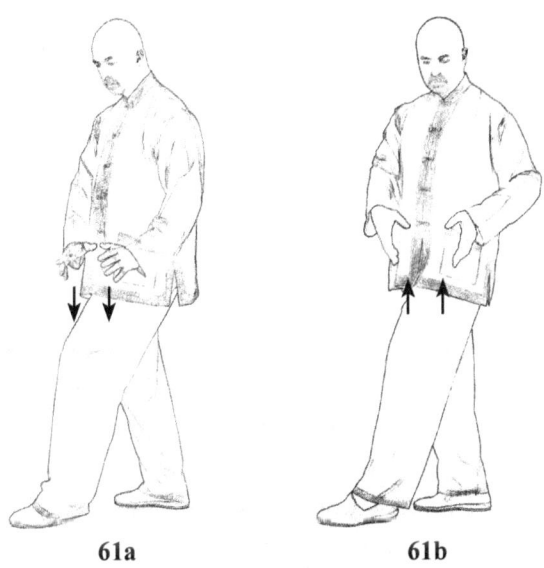

61a   61b

61a Facing the Western direction, gently move your bodyweight forward over the right leg and step forward with the left leg. The outer edge of the left foot (small toe) is just touching the ground. At the same time, look between the hands, with soft, relaxed fingers as if holding an egg, and the He Gu (web of hand) of both hands facing each other. Gently press down to the left in front of the Lower Dan Tian (area beneath the navel),

61b Raise the arms looking at the hands. Keep your fingers separated and relaxed and pointing to the ground as if softly picking up the egg. The fingers are slightly tense as they draw up the energy from the earth.

No. 2 to the middle

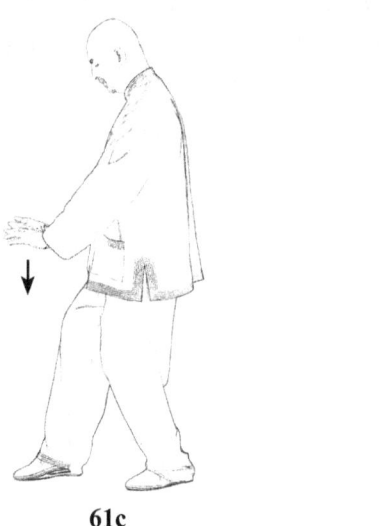
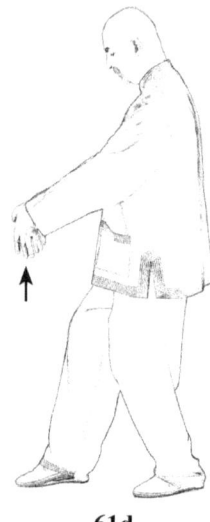

61c

61d

61c   Facing the Northern direction, gently move your bodyweight forward over the left leg and step forward with the right leg. The outer edge of the right foot (small toe) is just touching the ground. At the same time, look between the hands, with soft, relaxed fingers as if holding an egg, and the He Gu (web of hand) of both hands facing each other, gently press down in front of the Lower Dan Tian (area beneath the navel)

61d   Raise the arms looking at the hands. Keep your fingers separated and relaxed and pointing to the ground as if softly picking up the egg. The fingers are slightly tense as they draw up the energy from the earth.

No. 3 to the right

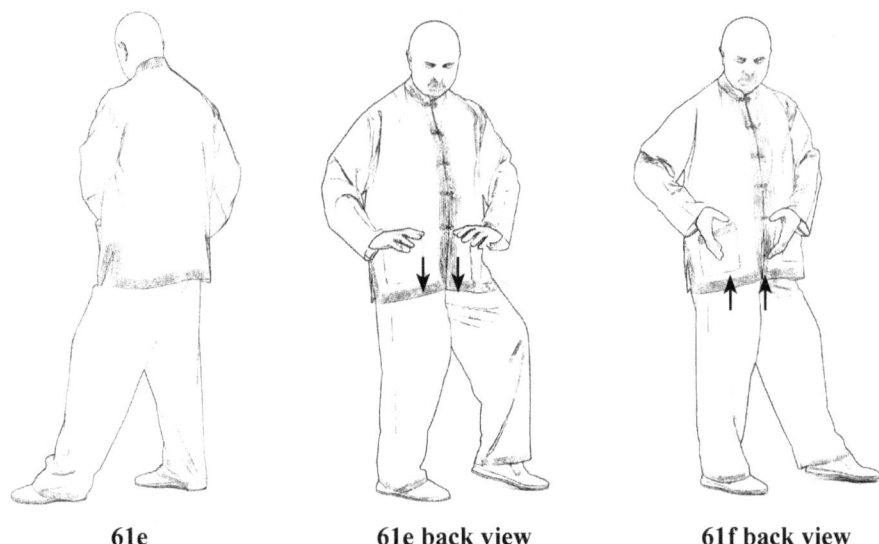

61e   61e back view   61f back view

61e   Facing the Eastern direction, gently move your bodyweight forward over the right leg and step forward with the left leg. The outer edge of the left foot (small toe) is just touching the ground. At the same time, look between the hands, with soft, relaxed fingers as if holding an egg, and the He Gu (web of hand) of both hands facing each other, gently press down to the right in front of the Lower Dan Tian (area beneath the navel).

61f   Raise the arms looking at the hands. Keep your fingers separated and relaxed and pointing to the ground as if softly picking up the egg. The fingers are slightly tense as they draw up the energy from the earth.

No. 4 to the right

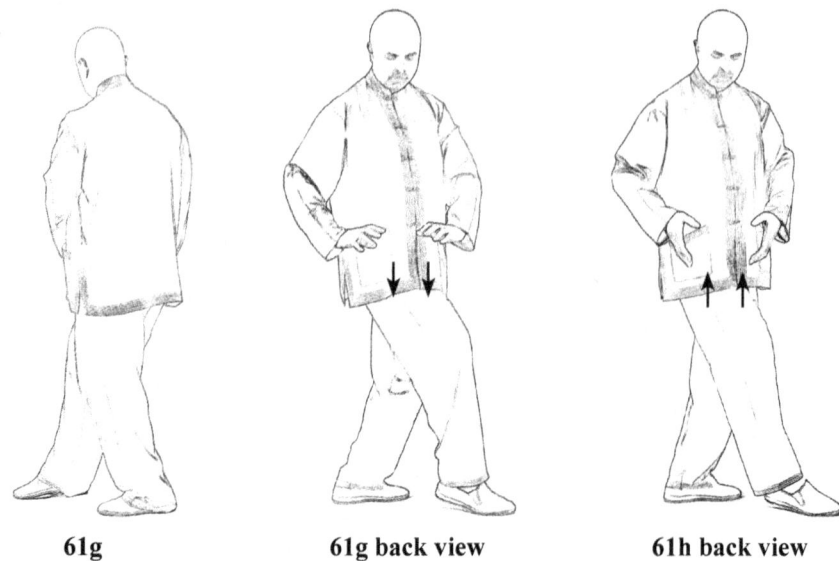

| 61g | 61g back view | 61h back view |

61g Facing the Eastern direction, gently move your bodyweight forward over the left leg and step forward with the right leg. The outer edge of the right foot (small toe) is just touching the ground. At the same time, look between the hands, with soft, relaxed fingers as if holding an egg, and the He Gu (web of hand) of both hands facing each other, gently press down to the right in front of the Lower Dan Tian (area beneath the navel).

61h Raise the arms looking at the hands. Keep your fingers separated and relaxed and pointing to the ground as if softly picking up the egg. The fingers are slightly tense as they draw up the energy from the earth.

No. 5 to the middle

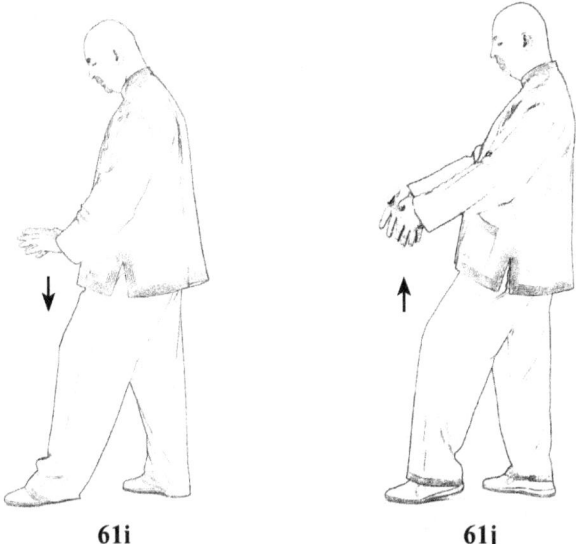

61i   **61j**

61i   Facing the Northern direction, gently move your bodyweight forward over the right leg and step forward with the left leg. The outer edge of the left foot (small toe) is just touching the ground. At the same time, look between the hands, with soft, relaxed fingers as if holding an egg, and the He Gu (web of hand) of both hands facing each other, gently press down in front of the Lower Dan Tian (area beneath the navel).

61j   Raise the arms looking at the hands. Keep your fingers separated and relaxed and pointing to the ground as if softly picking up the egg. The fingers are slightly tense as they draw up the energy from the earth.

No. 6 to the left

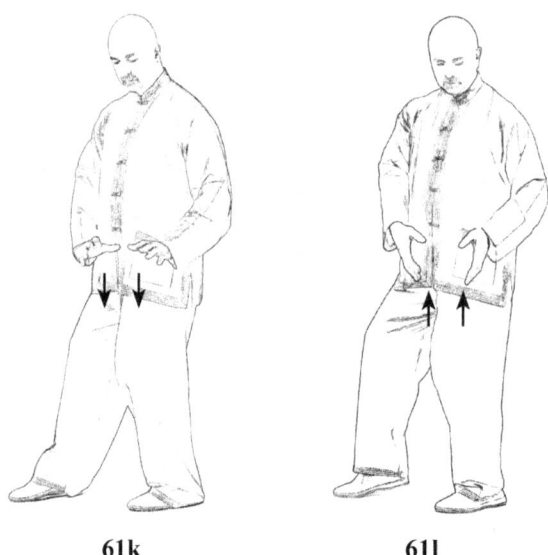

61k   61l

61k   Facing the Western direction, gently move your bodyweight forward over the left leg and step forward with the right leg. The outer edge of the right foot (small toe) is just touching the ground. At the same time, look between the hands, with soft, relaxed fingers as if holding an egg, and the He Gu (web of hand) of both hands facing each other, gently press down to the left in front of the Lower Dan Tian (area beneath the navel).

61L   Raise the arms looking at the hands. Keep your fingers separated and relaxed and pointing to the ground as if softly picking up the egg. The fingers are slightly tense as they draw up the energy from the earth.

No. 7 to the middle

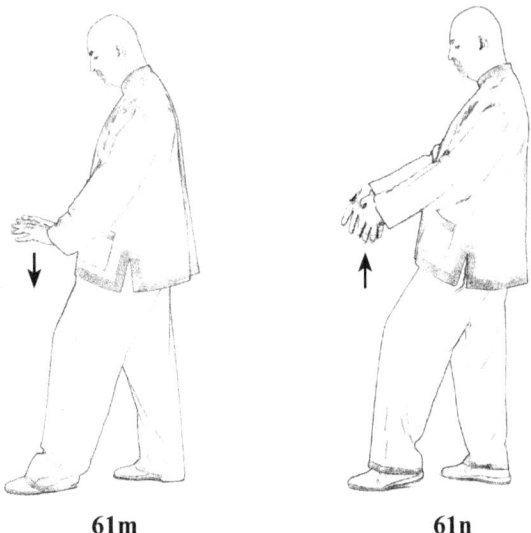

61m   61n

61m   Facing the Northern direction, gently move your bodyweight forward over the right leg and step forward with the left leg. The outer edge of the left foot (small toe) is just touching the ground. At the same time, look between the hands, with soft, relaxed fingers as if holding an egg, and the He Gu (web of hand) of both hands facing each other, gently press down in front of the Lower Dan Tian (area beneath the navel).

61n   Raise the arms looking at the hands. Keep your fingers separated and relaxed and pointing to the ground as if softly picking up the egg. The fingers are slightly tense as they draw up the energy from the earth.

62. Turning the body and fluttering the wings 转身 泳动

The bodyweight remains on the right leg after the seventh 'Looking for the nest' movement.

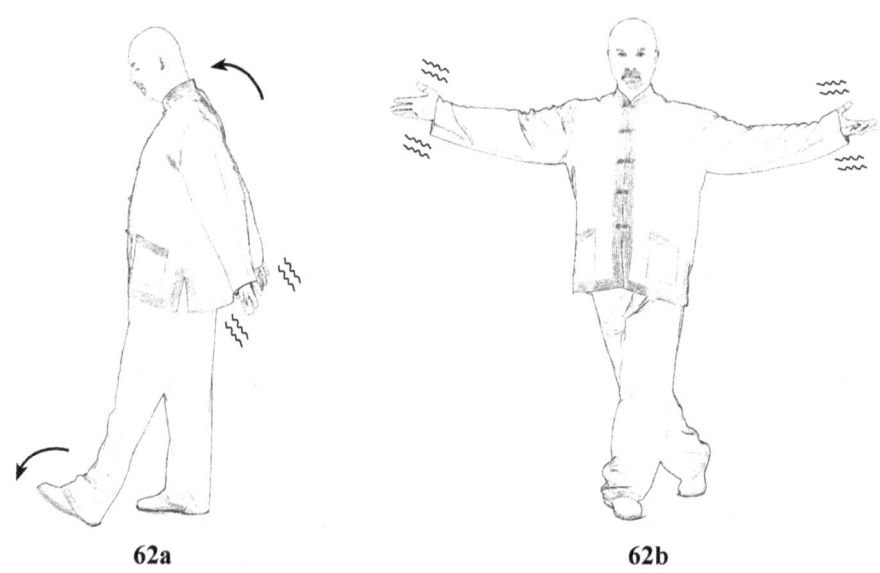

62a   **62b**

62a Relax the wrists and hands and gently start to flutter the arms with the palms facing backward. Move fluttering arms back to the side of the body level with the hips. At the same time, move your bodyweight back onto the right leg and lift the left toe.

62b Raise both fluttering arms up to shoulder height with the palms facing up and turn the left foot 90° counter clockwise. Move your bodyweight on to the left foot, turn the body from the waist turning 90° and cross the legs to face the Western direction.

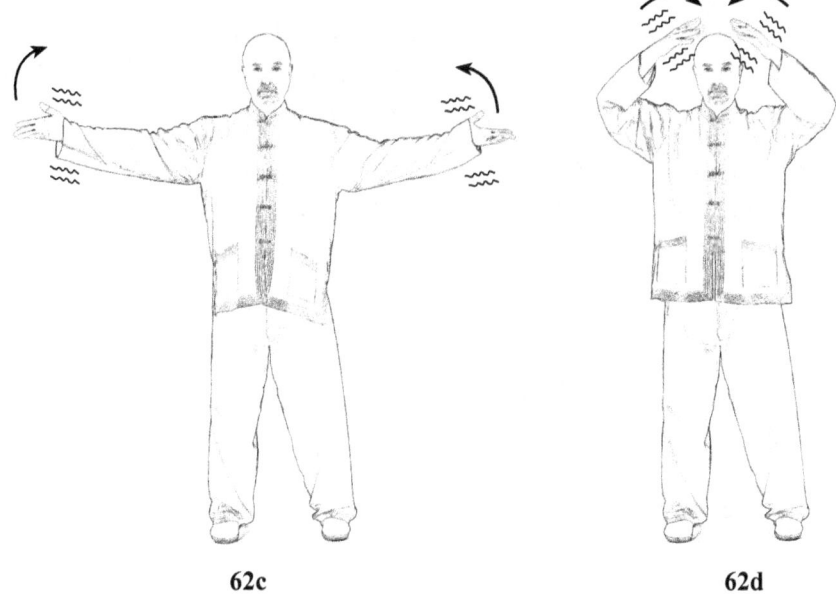

62c   **62d**

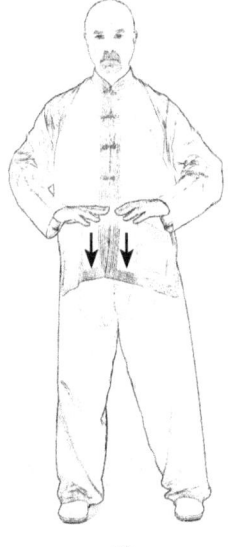

62c Step around with your right leg so both feet are parallel at about shoulder-width apart. Move your bodyweight forward over the balls of your feet lifting both heels slightly off the ground.

62d,e Raise fluttering arms up over your forehead keeping shoulders relaxed and guiding Qi to the top of the head. Lower your arms with palms facing the body and slowly reduce the fluttering. Your fingers are pointing down at the Lower Dan Tian (area beneath the navel).

62e

63.   Sleeping peacefully and recovering the Qi 安睡归气

This movement brings the refined Qi to the Lower Dan Tian (area beneath the navel) and stimulates the Heavenly Orbit. It is important to keep a quiet mind during this movement as it is a type of meditation.

Stay in this position for 10-60 seconds. Find a position that is comfortable - any comfortable position has benefits. If you find that you lose your balance, simply keep your eyes open.

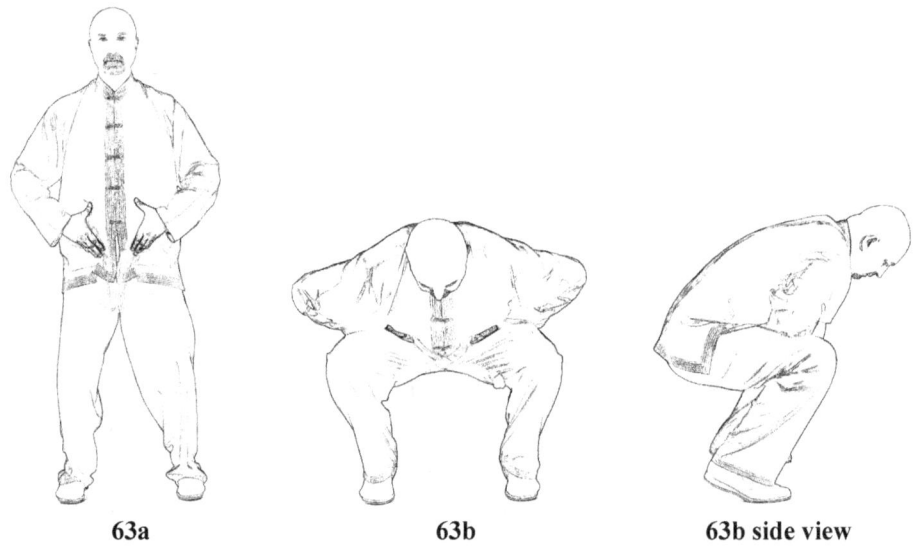

63a   63b   63b side view

63a   Turn your fingers into the Dai Mai (Gall Bladder GB26) at the side of the body below the 11th rib at the same height as the navel with thumbs on Ru Gen (Stomach ST18) beneath the middle of the ribs which is the 5th intercostal space just below the nipple.

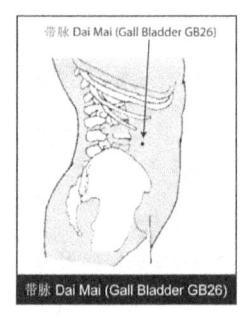

63b   Squat down with your bodyweight over the balls of your feet lifting both heels off the ground. Both palms are around the abdominal area and fingers are gently pressing into the groin. This allows Qi to settle at the Lower Dan Tian (area beneath the navel). The eyes are closed. Stay in this resting position for 10-60 seconds.

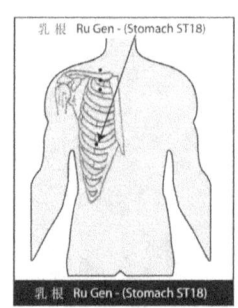

64. Closing movement 收式

Slowly open your eyes and lift your head looking to the front. Place heels on the ground and very gently raise your body. The arms are in a natural position to the side.

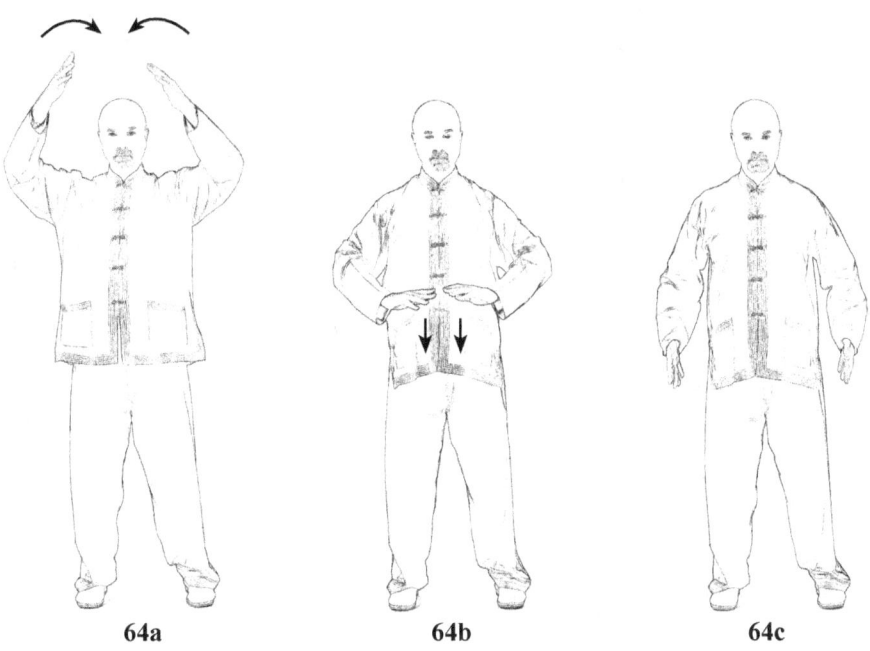

64a   64b   64c

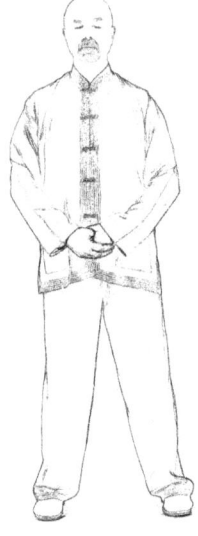

64a,b,c Lift arms up over your head, keeping the shoulders relaxed. Guide Qi to the top of the head, to the chest and to the Lower Dan Tian (area beneath the navel). Repeat a total of three times.

64d The tip of your right thumb touches the left Lao Gong (middle of palm); relax the hands and fingers. The hands make a Yin Yang shape. Place your hands over the Lower Dan Tian (area beneath the navel) and close the eyes in meditation.

64d

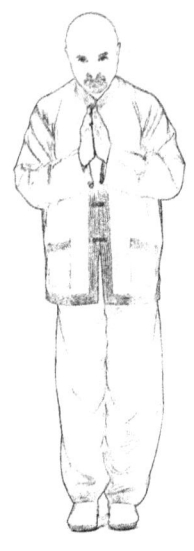

Close with meditation

After practising the dynamic moving sections of the Da Yan Wild Goose Qigong, we practise the static or stillness section. This part of our practice is very important; when the body comes to a complete stop, the Qi keeps moving and through the tranquillity of the mind, the Qi will come into order. It's what we call the 'processing' stage; it's important to keep your thinking mind out of the way and to allow the Qi to do its work.

The final stage is ideally fifteen minutes of meditation, either sitting cross-legged on the floor or on the edge of a chair keeping the back straight. The chin is tucked in, with the tip of the tongue on the top palate of the mouth, just behind the teeth. Breathe naturally in and out through the nose. Sensing the breath and sensing the peace. Allow the breath to become smooth and even and the mind to rest for at least five minutes. Turn the hands in over the Dan Tian, the area beneath the navel, with one hand on top of the other. Allow your mind, breath and energy to settle. When breathing in, the abdomen gently pushes out into your hands. When breathing out gently push the hands in. Relax and feel the whole body breathe for another five minutes. After the face rubbing routine (on the next page), place the hands with palms down on the knees sensing the inner peace. Through the peace, allow the heart to open like a smile, with a wave of loving kindness permeating from the heart through the whole body. Just relax and let it go out through every cell. Every cell of the body is smiling with the radiance of the universe as you become one with the universe for another five minutes.

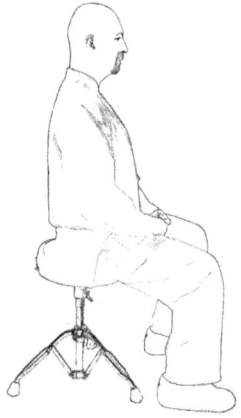
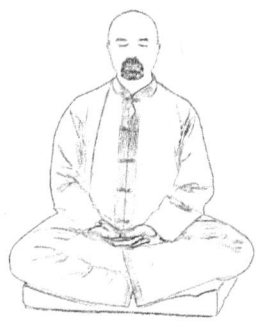

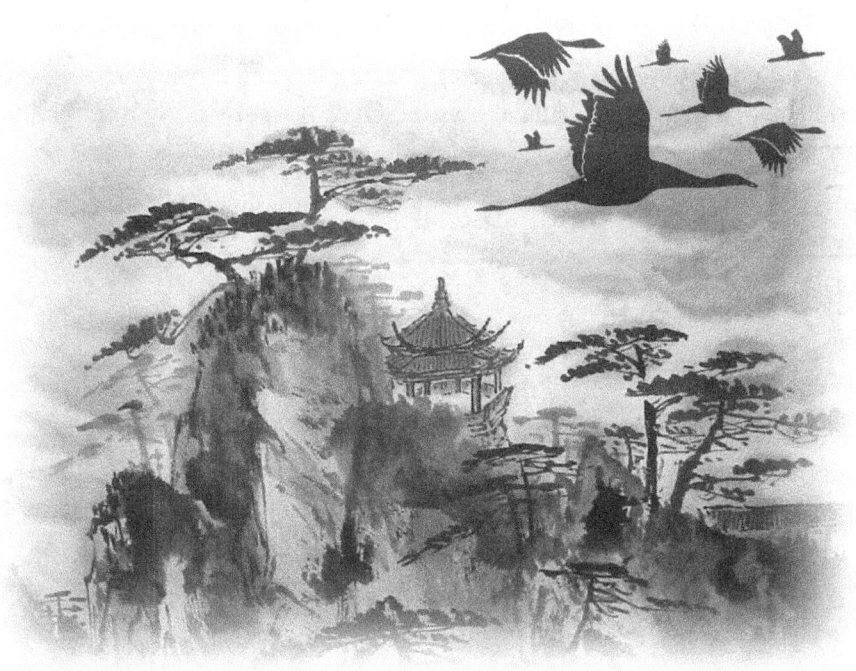

Chapter 8

Gathering the Qi and Rubbing the Face

Da Yan - Wild Goose Qigong
The 1st 64 movements

Gathering the Qi and Rubbing the Face

The practice of Qigong helps clear the energy channels and dredges the meridians of stagnant Qi. This allows the Qi to flow smoothly through the body and creates an energy or Qi field.

We generally feel this Qi field in the hands. To gather and refine the Qi move the hands in and out as follows:

Gathering the Qi

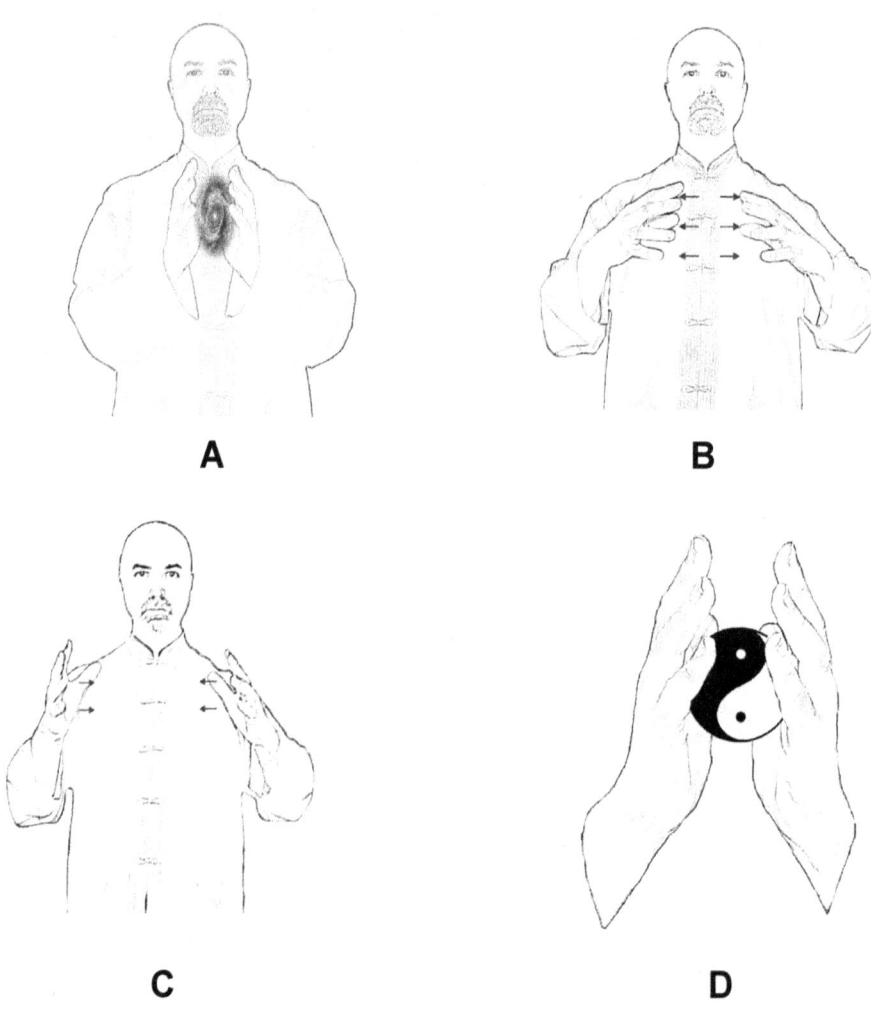

A

B

C

D

A Hold the hands in front of the body at chest height as if holding a ball of energy or light.

B Slightly draw the hands away from each other tensing the fingers.

C Then push the hands closer compressing the Qi between the hands.

Repeat six times.

D Relax and feel. We will generally feel warmth, like a field of energy between the hands. This creates a polarity as the left hand is Yang (positive) and the right hand is Yin (negative).

Now that the hands are charged with Qi it's a time for healing by placing the hands on a sore or injured part of your body or by massaging the face. Your face has many meridian acupuncture points that connect the meridians to the internal organs.

Face rubbing

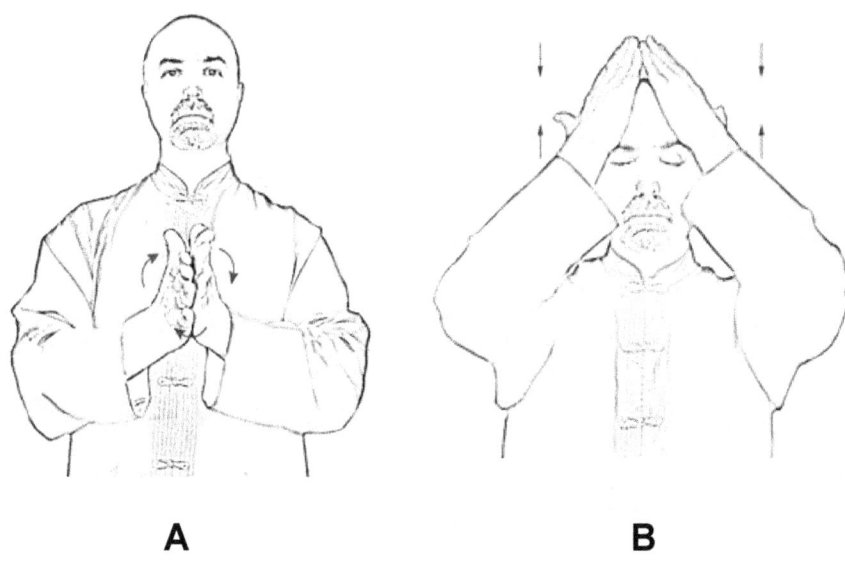

A   **B**

A Rub the hands together and bring the healing energy through your heart into your hands.

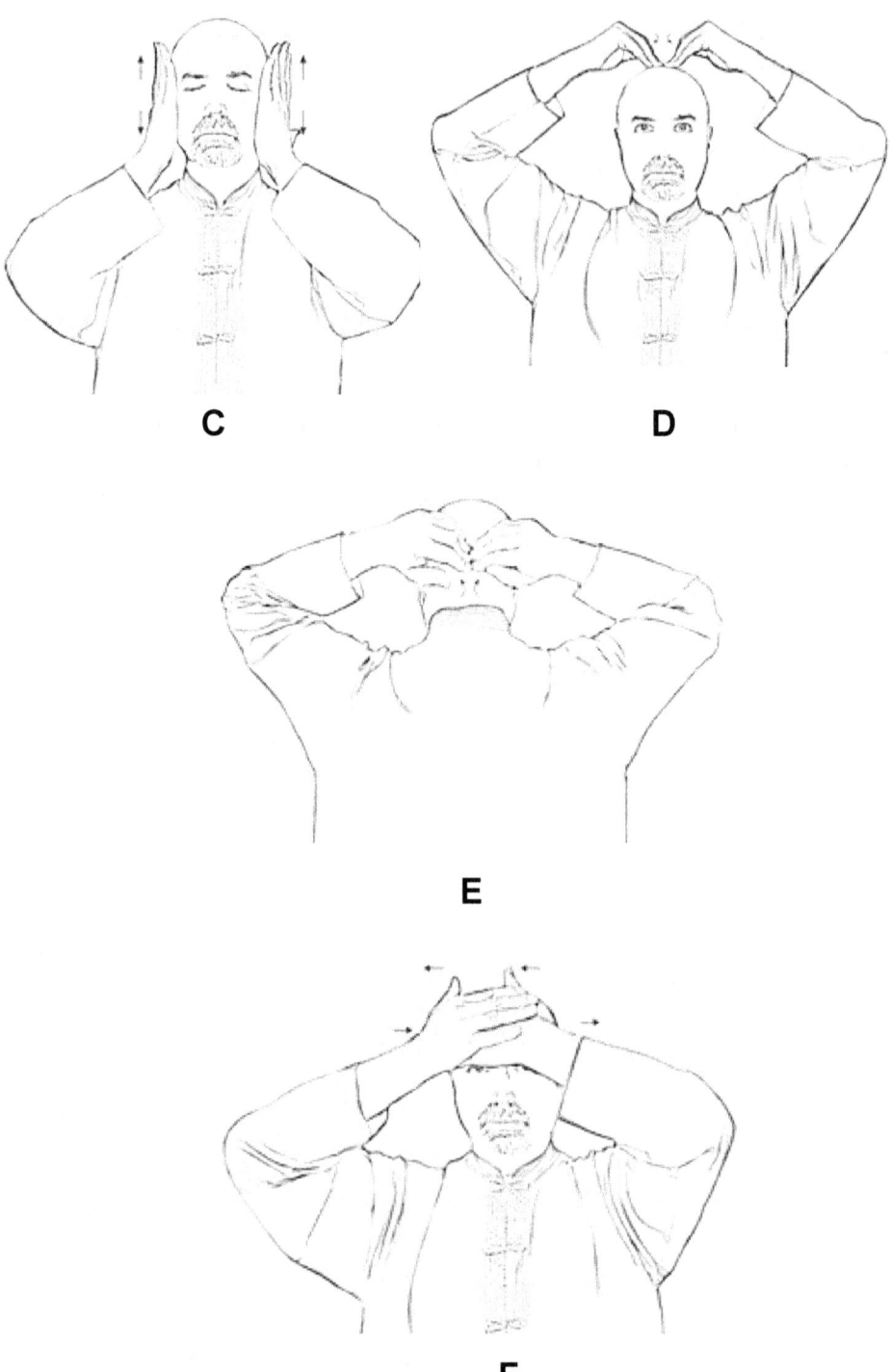

C

D

E

F

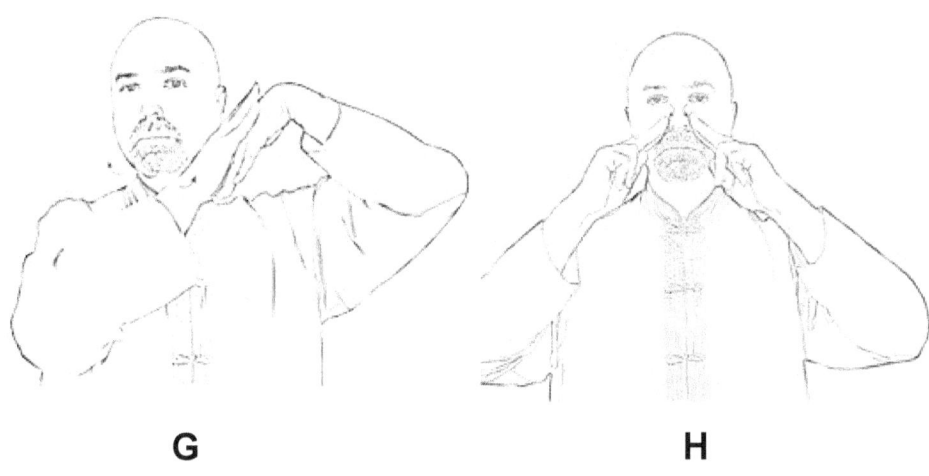

G

H

B, C Place the warm palms over your eyes (liver). Feel the warmth going in. Then rub the hands up and down from the forehead to the chin, the side of the face, then around the eyes and cheeks in a circular motion, like washing the face.

Rub around the ears with the tip of the fingers massaging around the outside of the ears down to the ear lobe. With the tips of the fingers, massage around the inside of the ear following all the grooves, stimulating the kidneys.

D, E With the tips of the fingers, massage back through the hair and then rub the back of the neck. Gently massage the base of the skull, the top of the head and massage up over the head and scalp.

F, G, H With one hand on top of the other rub the palm across the forehead and then rub around the chin letting the knuckles massage the jaw. Rub the fingers down the sides of the nose and around the cheek bones (lung).

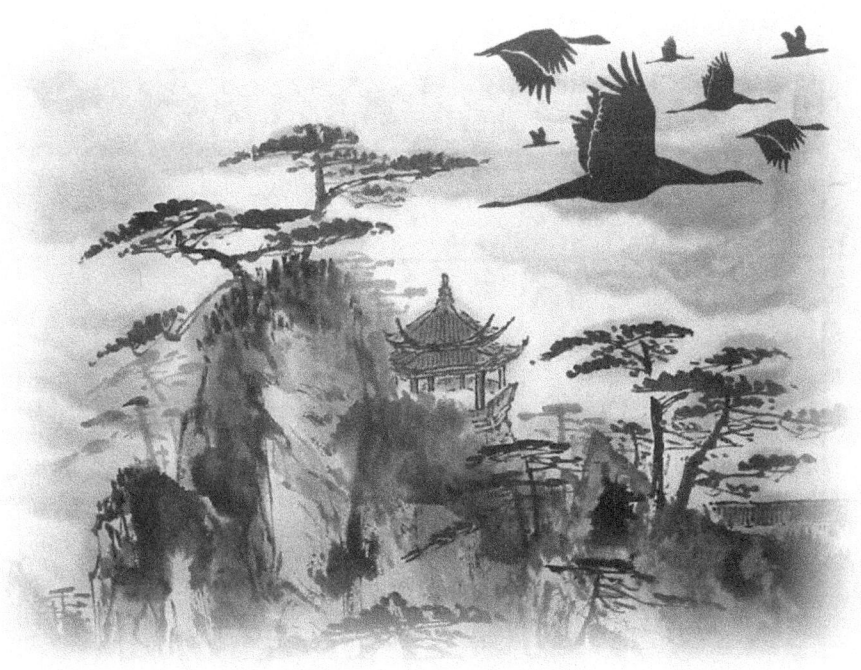

Chapter 9

Meridian Charts

Da Yan - Wild Goose Qigong
The 1st 64 movements

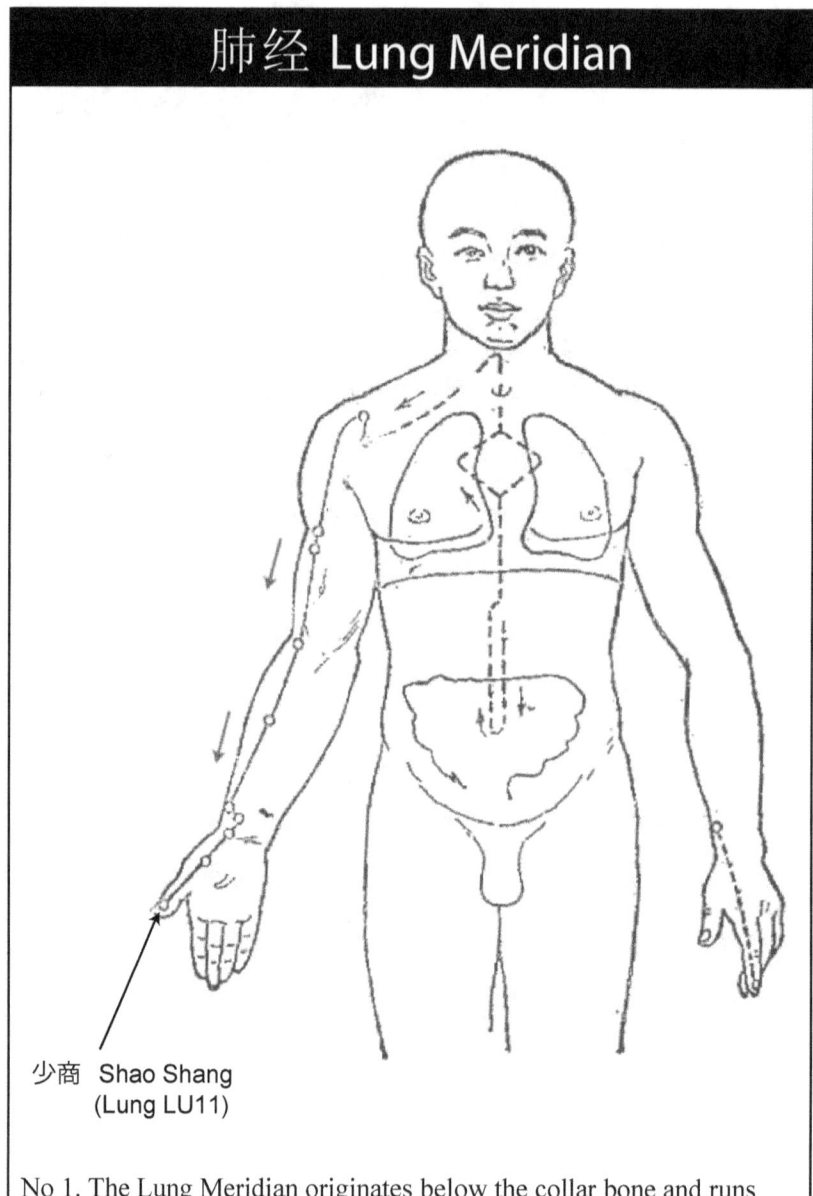

少商 Shao Shang
(Lung LU11)

No 1. The Lung Meridian originates below the collar bone and runs down the inside of the arm to the outside of the thumb.

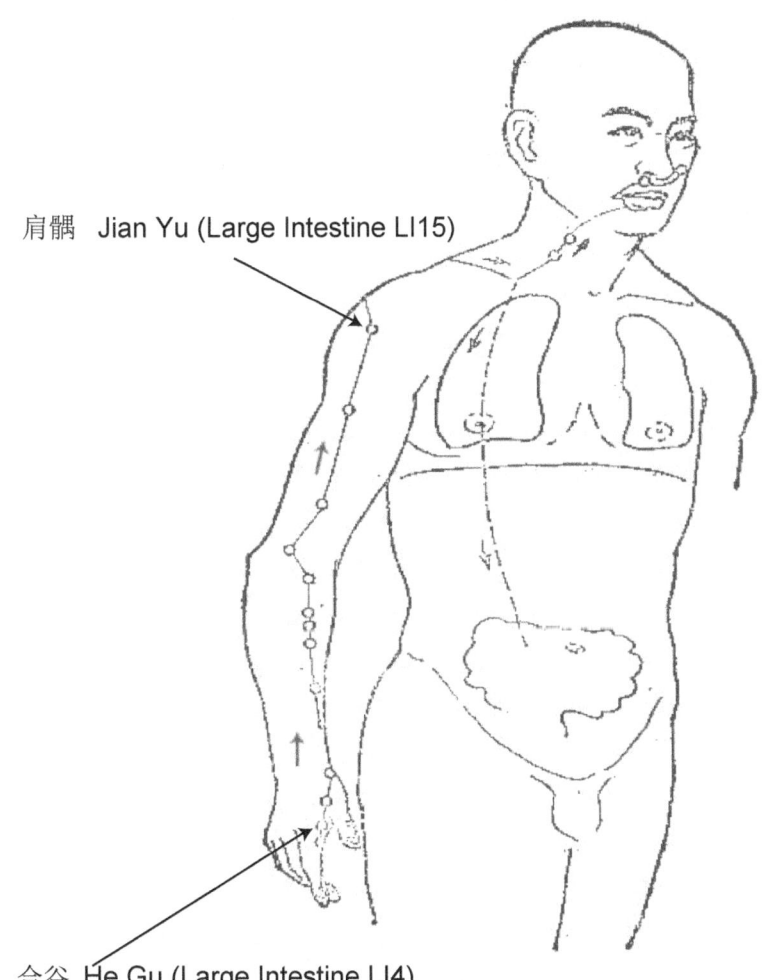

肩髃　Jian Yu (Large Intestine LI15)

合谷 He Gu (Large Intestine LI4)

No 2. The Large Intestine Meridian (Yang) originates from the outside of the index finger through the He Gu, along the outside of the arm to the shoulder, to the neck and finishes on the opposite side of the face near the nose and cheek bone.

脾经 Spleen Meridian

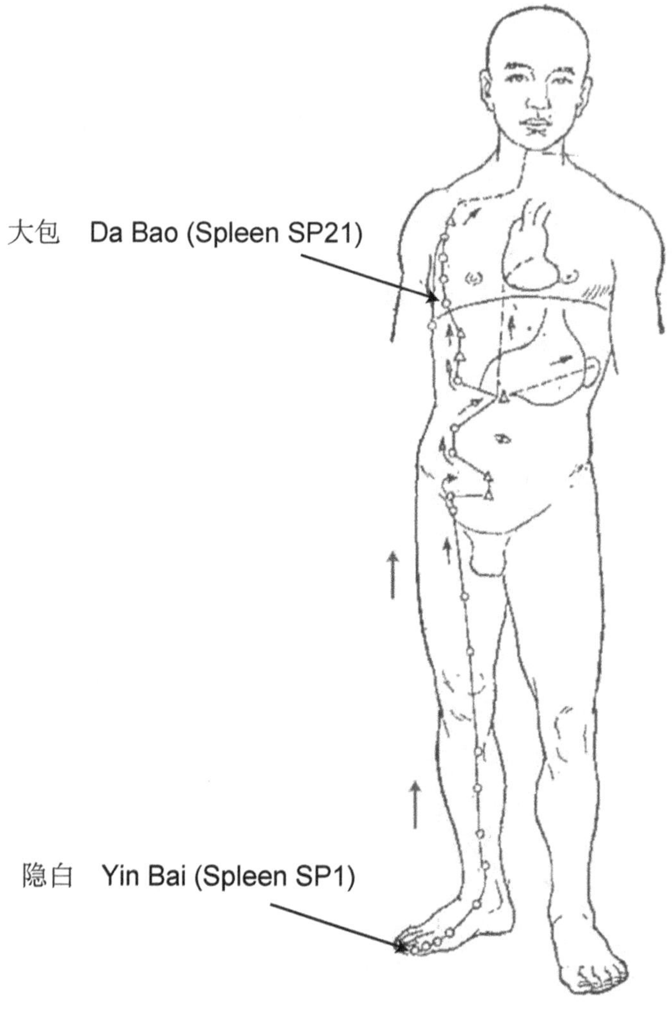

大包　Da Bao (Spleen SP21)

隐白　Yin Bai (Spleen SP1)

No 3. The Spleen Meridian (Yin) originates from the outside of the big toe, and rises up past the ankle the inside of the leg to the hip, through the abdomen to the chest and up to the oesophagus and under the tongue.

胃经 Stomach Meridian

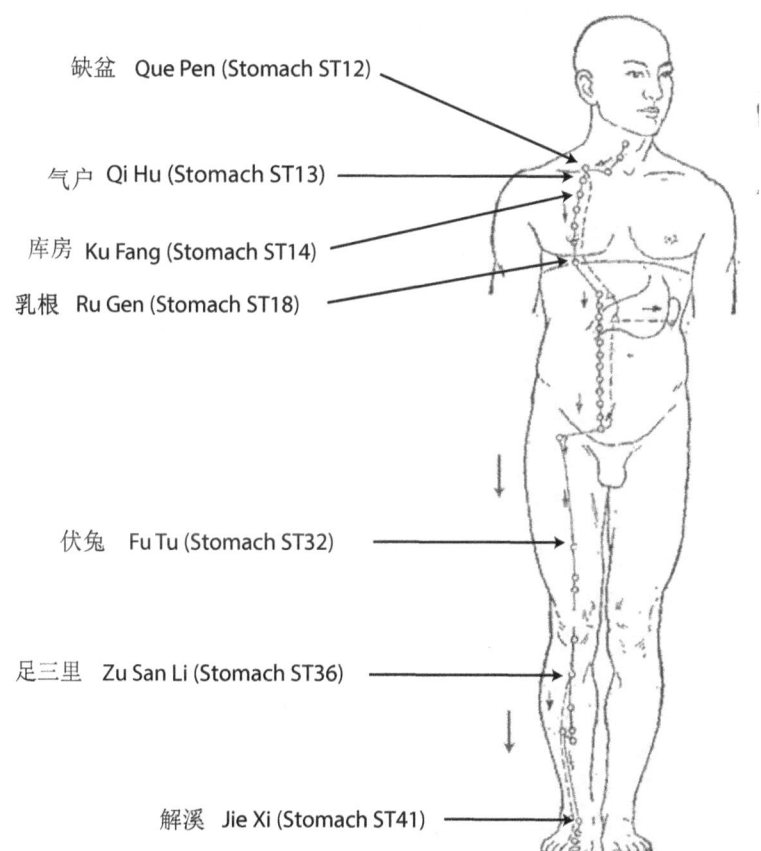

缺盆 Que Pen (Stomach ST12)

气户 Qi Hu (Stomach ST13)

库房 Ku Fang (Stomach ST14)

乳根 Ru Gen (Stomach ST18)

伏兔 Fu Tu (Stomach ST32)

足三里 Zu San Li (Stomach ST36)

解溪 Jie Xi (Stomach ST41)

No 4. The Stomach Meridian (Yang) originates from beneath the eye, down to the corner of the mouth, around the jaw, down the neck to the nipple, and down the body to the pubic bone. It then continues down the front of the leg to the front of the ankle and finishes on the outside of the second toe.

肝经 Liver Meridian

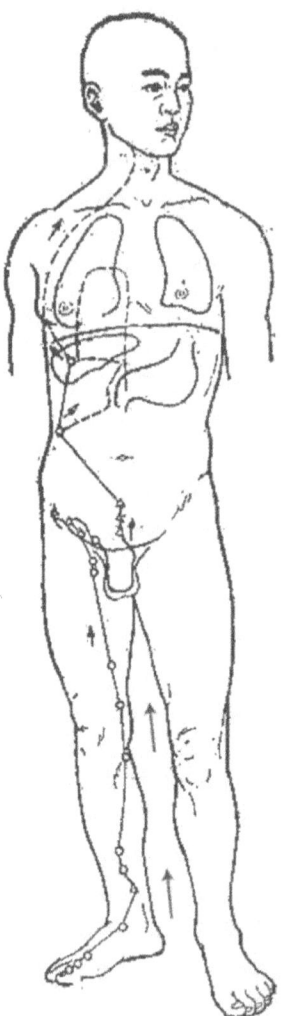

No 5. The Liver Meridian (Yin) originates from the inside of the big toe, rises up the inside of the leg into the body past the hip, and finishes at the lower rib area.

胆经 Gall Bladder Meridian

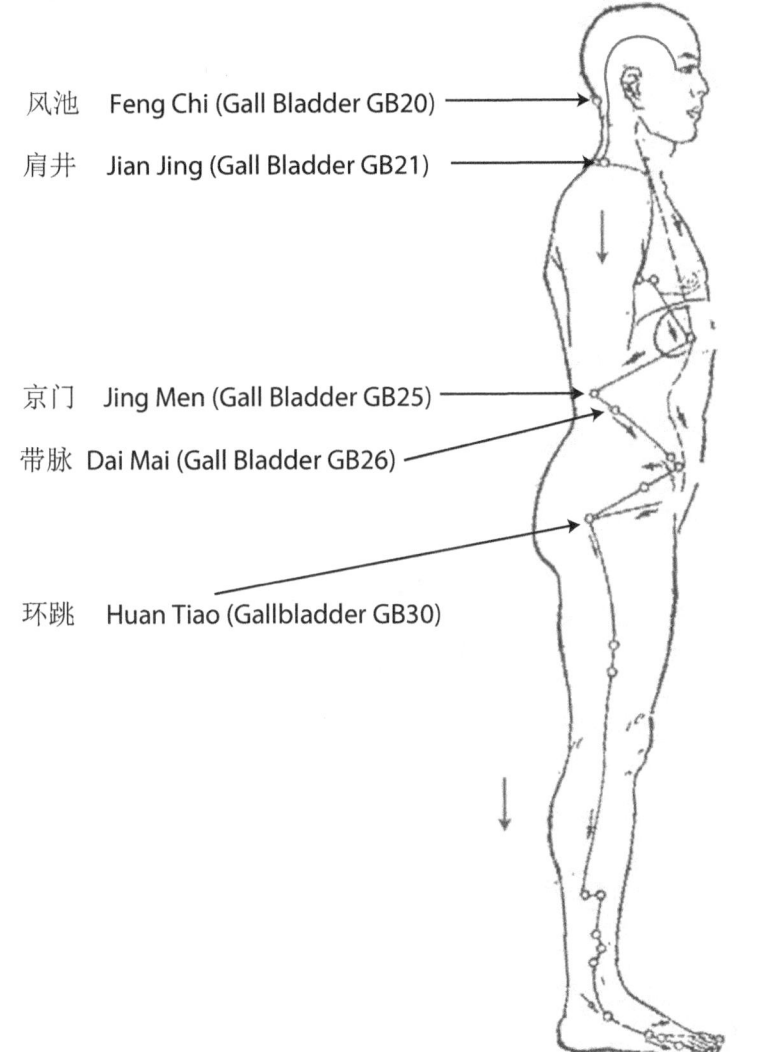

风池 Feng Chi (Gall Bladder GB20)

肩井 Jian Jing (Gall Bladder GB21)

京门 Jing Men (Gall Bladder GB25)

带脉 Dai Mai (Gall Bladder GB26)

环跳 Huan Tiao (Gallbladder GB30)

No 6. The Gall Bladder Meridian (Yang) originates from the outer corner of the eye, runs around the ear, down the neck, under the arm and down the side of the body, the outside of the leg, the outside of the foot and finishes at the outside of the fourth toe.

肾经 Kidney Meridian

涌泉　Yong Quan (Kidney K1)

No 7. The Kidney Meridian (Yin) originates from the sole of the foot and rises up the inside of the leg, through the abdomen to the collar bone.

膀胱经 Urinary Bladder Meridian

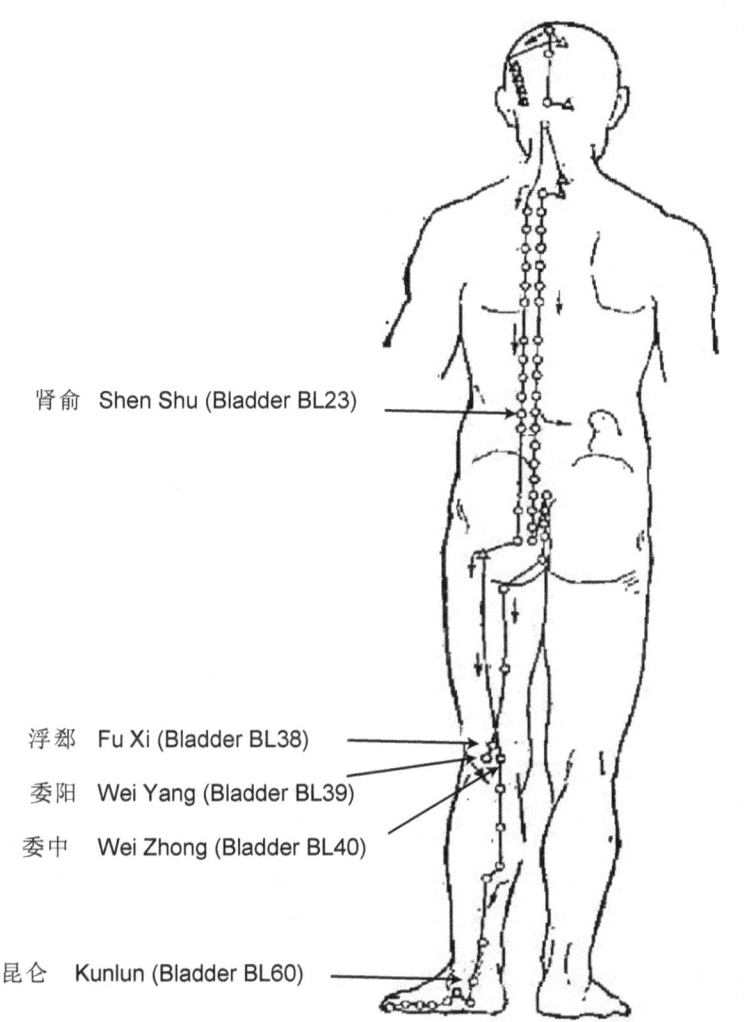

肾俞 Shen Shu (Bladder BL23)

浮郄 Fu Xi (Bladder BL38)

委阳 Wei Yang (Bladder BL39)

委中 Wei Zhong (Bladder BL40)

昆仑 Kunlun (Bladder BL60)

No 8. The Bladder Meridian (Yang) originates near the eyebrow and goes back over the head, down the back to the hip, the back of the legs to the heel, then along the outside of the foot finishing on the outside of the small toe.

心 经 Heart Meridian

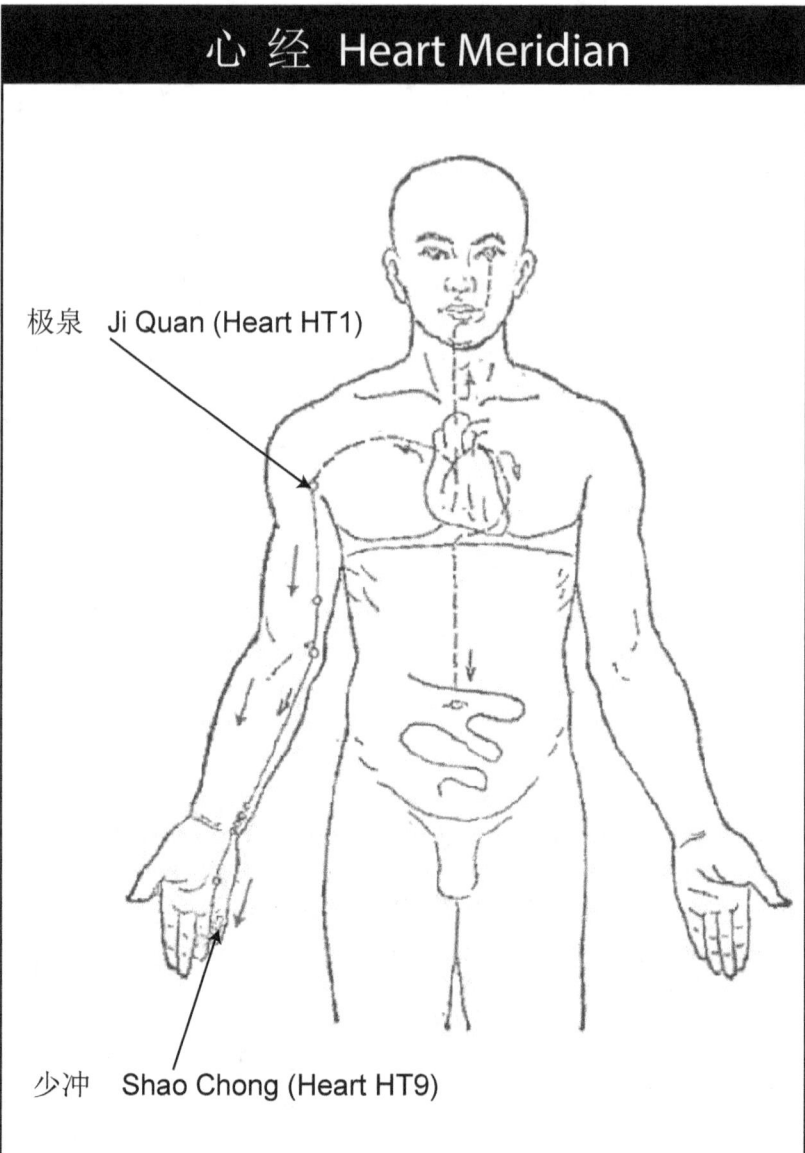

极泉 Ji Quan (Heart HT1)

少冲 Shao Chong (Heart HT9)

No 9. The Heart Meridian (Yin) originates from the armpit, past the elbow to the outside of the wrist finishing at the end of the inside of the small finger.

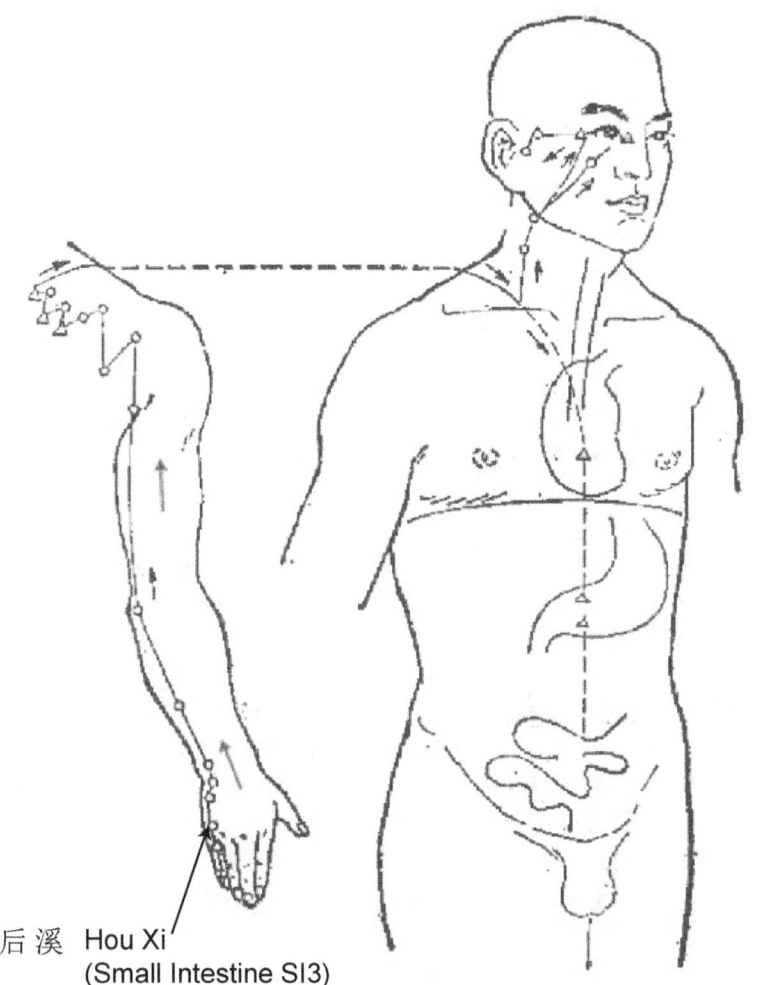

小肠经 Small Intestine Meridian

后溪 Hou Xi
(Small Intestine SI3)

No 10. The Small Intestine Meridian (Yang) originates from the outside tip of the little finger and runs along the outside of the arm to the shoulder, then to the neck and cheek and finishes near the ear at the depression created when the mouth is opened.

心包经 Pericardium Meridian

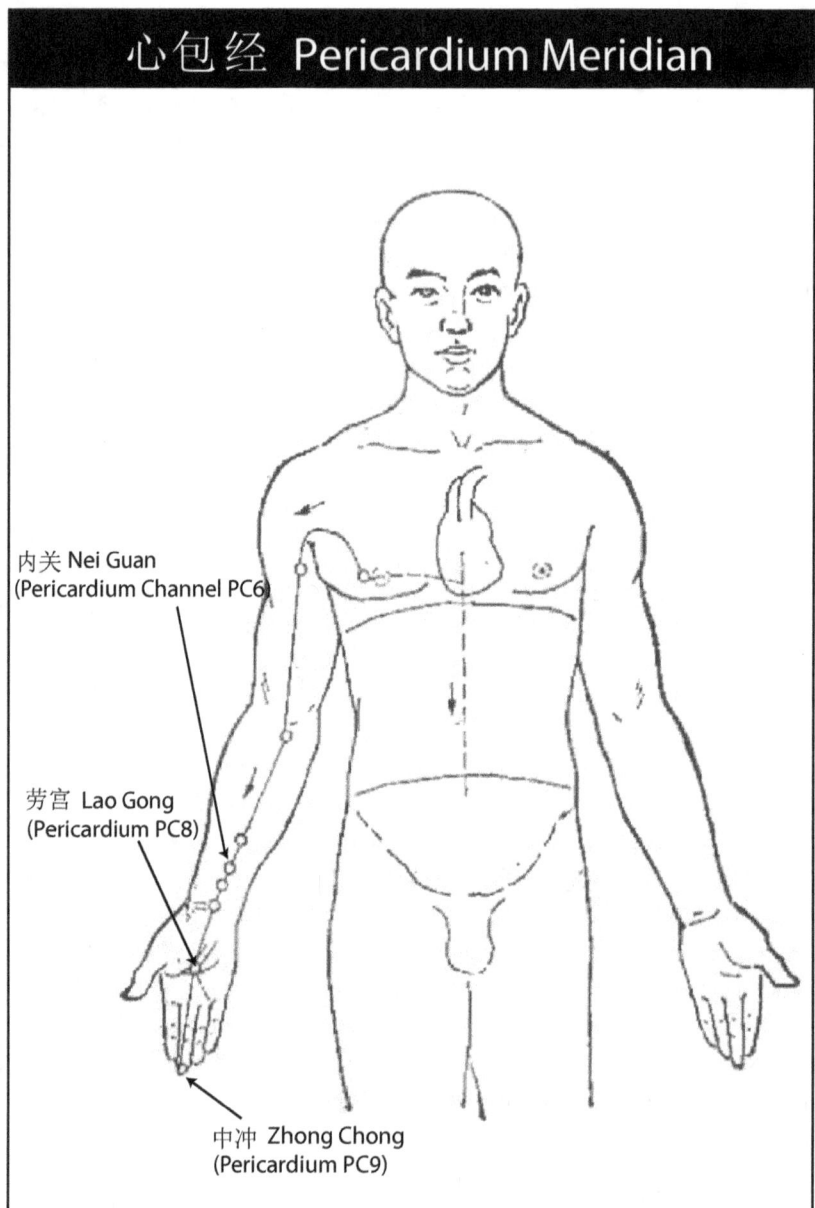

内关 Nei Guan
(Pericardium Channel PC6)

劳宫 Lao Gong
(Pericardium PC8)

中冲 Zhong Chong
(Pericardium PC9)

No 11. The Pericardium Meridian (Yin) originates next to the nipple and flows down the centre of the inside of the arm, finishing at the middle finger.

三焦经　Triple warmer Meridian

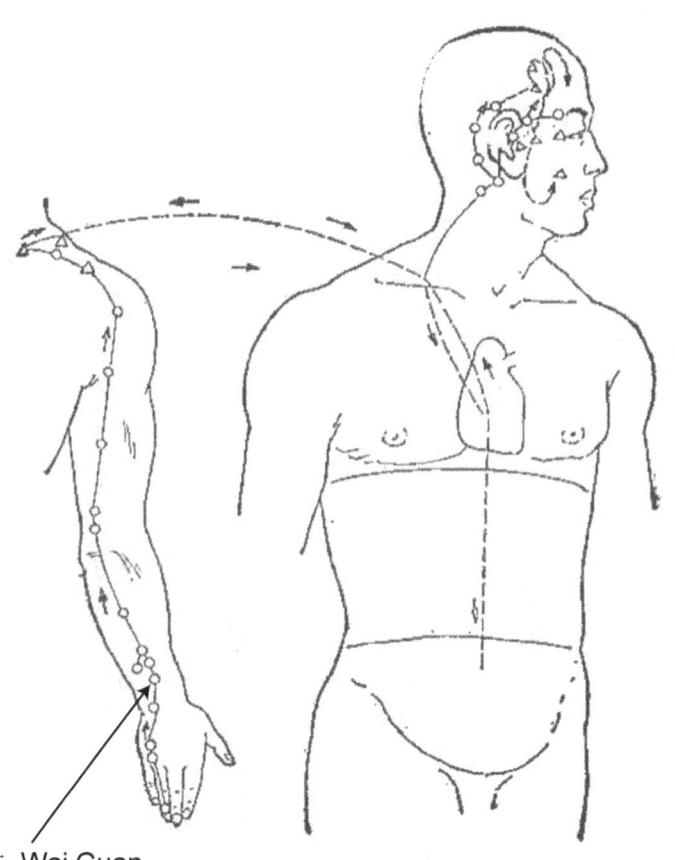

外关 Wai Guan
(Triple Burner Channel TE5)

No 12. The Triple Burner Meridian (Yang) starts at the tip of the ring finger, rises up the outside of the arm, the back of the shoulder to the collarbone, up the outside of the neck, and behind the ear before it dips down to the cheek and ends under the eye. An internal branch descends into the chest, through the diaphragm to the abdomen

督脉 Du Channel

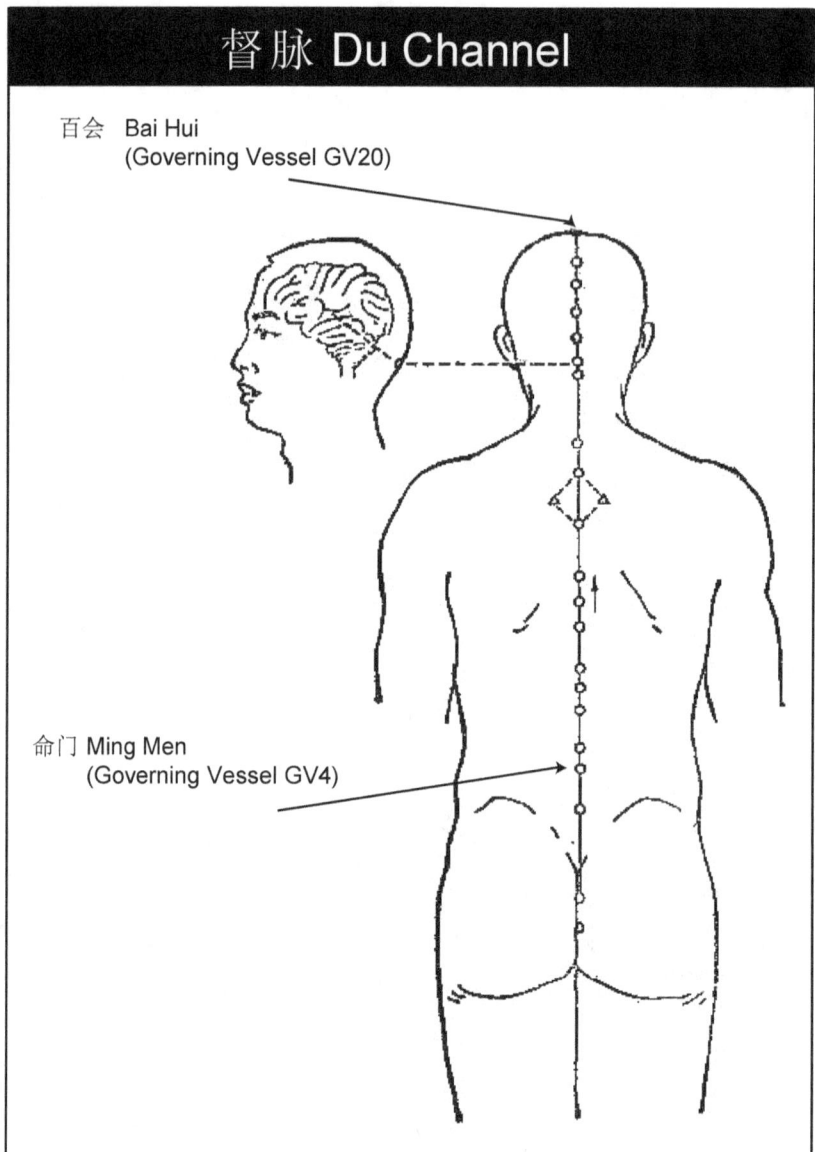

百会　Bai Hui
(Governing Vessel GV20)

命门 Ming Men
(Governing Vessel GV4)

No 1. The Du Channel runs from the anus, up the spine and across the crown of the head to finish inside the upper lip.

任脉 Ren Channel

气海 Qi Hai
(Conception Vessel CV6)

Hui Yin

No 2. The Ren Channel originates in the uterus in females and in the lower abdomen in males and emerges at the Hui Yin in the perineum. It moves up the middle of the abdomen to the jaw, ending just below the lower lip.

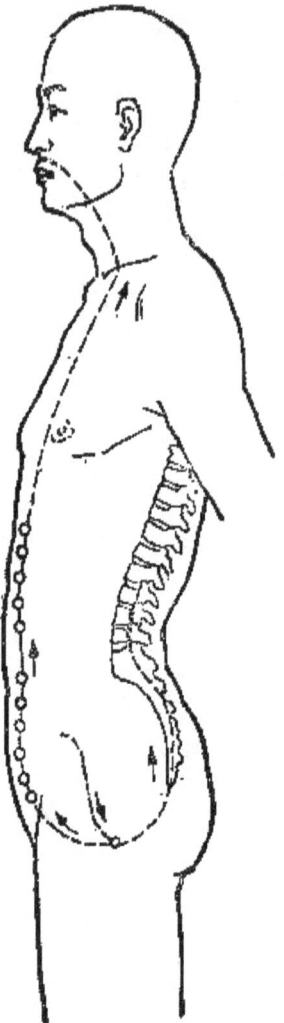

No 3. The Chong Channel originates from inside the body to the perineum then ascends through the spine, the channel braches out along both sides of the abdomen up to the throat and finishing around the lips.

带 脉 Dai Channel

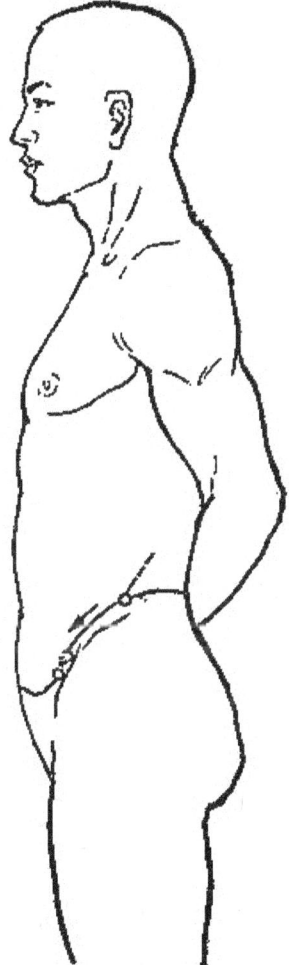

No 4. The Dai Channel (Girdle Vessel) runs around the waist like a belt.

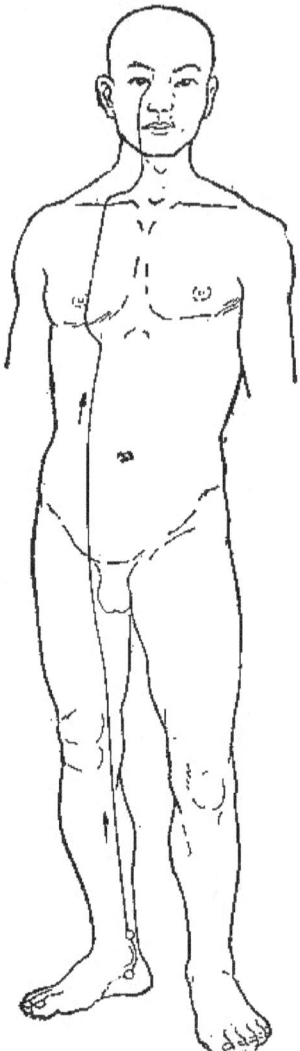

No 5. The Yin Qiao Channel travels along the inside of the heel and the leg, up the abdomen and the chest to the top of the collarbone. It passes along the throat, by the side of the mouth and nose, to the inner edge of the eye.

阳跷脉 Yang Qiao Channel

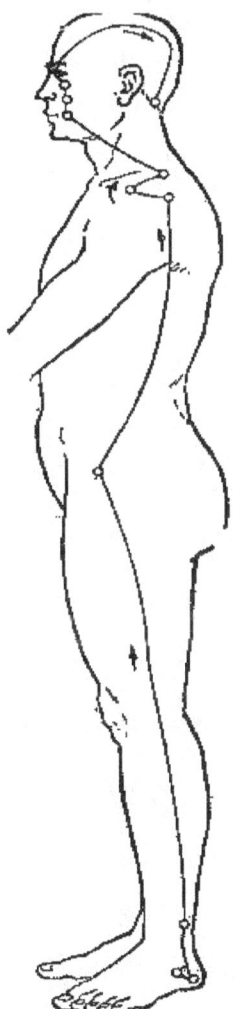

No 6. The Yang Qiao Channel, travels up the outside of the leg from the heel, to the thigh, the armpit, through the back of the shoulder and ascends the neck to the corner of the mouth, then passing over the head to finish at the nape of the neck.

阴维脉 Yin Wei Channel

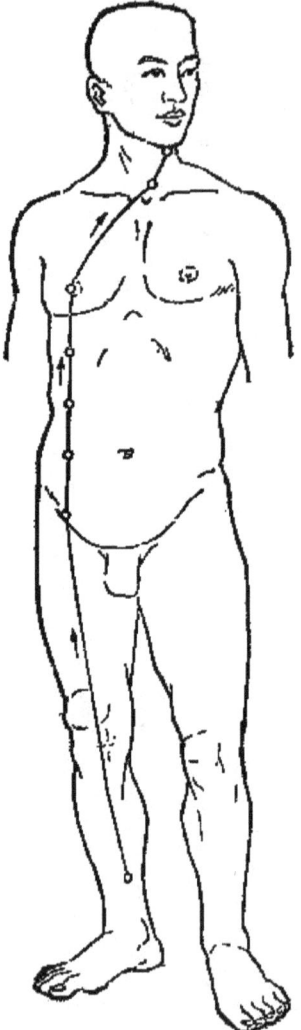

No 7. The Yin Wei Channel originates at the front of the leg, travels through the hip, over the chest and ends in the neck on the opposite side.

阳维脉 Yang Wei Channel

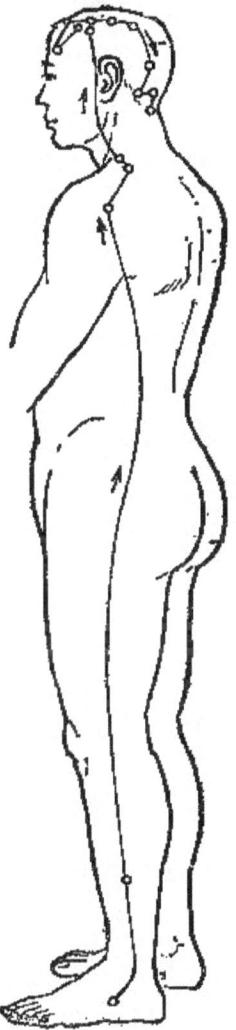

No 8. The Yang Wei Channel originates on the outside of the heel, moving up the outside of the leg to the hip, armpit, shoulder and neck. It then moves upwards to the cheeks and forehead then turns backwards to the back of the neck.

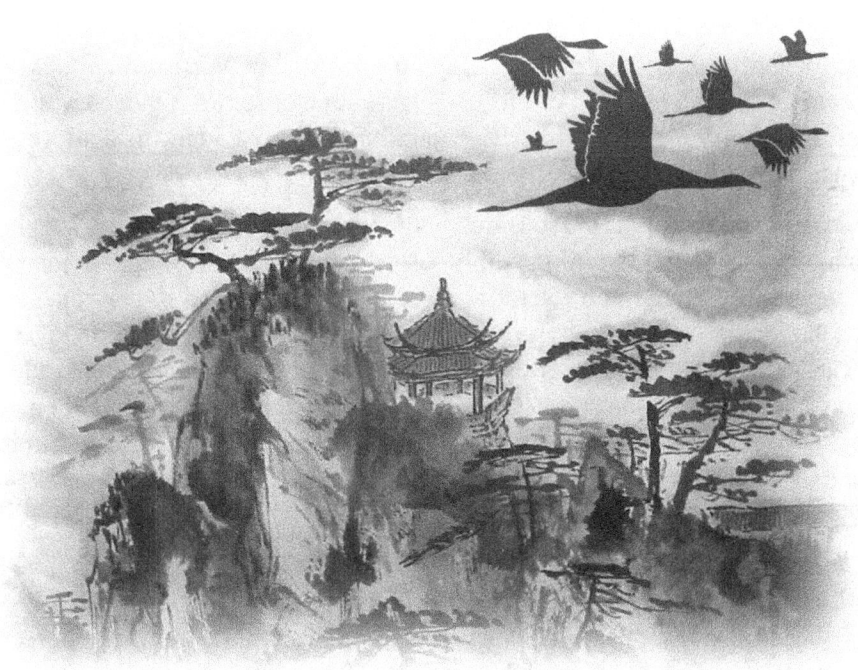

Chapter 10

Stories to Inspire

Da Yan - Wild Goose Qigong
The 1st 64 movements

Stories to Inspire:

I first began to learn and practise Qigong after recovering from an episode of pneumonia that had landed me in hospital. I recognised that my busy stressful work and lifestyle at that time had contributed, so I sought to achieve some balance in my life.

I had attended several of Simon Blow's Qigong retreats at Sunnataram Thai Forest Monastery and found them incredibly restoring and beneficial and so jumped at the opportunity to attend a retreat there specifically devoted to Da Yan. I really liked the idea of applying myself wholeheartedly to learn a new form. That first Da Yan Wild Goose Qigong retreat was the first of many more that I have attended at Sunnataram, Bruarong and in China. Da Yan is such a beautiful form to practise in a group and the more I learn and practise this form, the more I gain from it and love it.

I have been very fortunate to spend time learning Da Yan Gong with Master Chen in China in the summers of 2011 and 2012. What a privilege to spend time with and learn from this very great but humble, cheerful man who is so full of life and energy. Learning from Master Chen is so special because he is directly descended from those who first developed this ancient art. His energy is truly palpable. He is passionate about maintaining the form true to the teachings he has received and his passion is contagious!

Qigong is the practice of working with the energy of the body, by way of mindful movement, mindfulness of thinking (or non-thinking) and mindfulness of breathing.

Practising Qigong makes me feel whole and in spiritual balance. I move more smoothly and am stronger and more flexible when I practise. I feel connected internally with the earth and with the universe. I always feel very connected to and grateful to my teachers when I practise. To me Qigong is akin to a universal prayer. I am calmer and more mindful when I practise regularly and so more able to respond to others' needs in a helpful way.

Qigong helps me to feel whole, in balance, connected and fluid, rather than stilted. Of all the forms I have learned I have found Da Yan to be the most beneficial. I feel so well physically, emotionally and spiritually when I practise Da Yan regularly. I understand what matters is this moment right here and now. Experience this moment without expectation and allow nothingness.

Thank you Simon for all the time and effort you have put in to enable us to experience Da Yan Gong through Master Chen and for the tremendous work you are doing to keep Da Yan true and accurate to his teachings.

Fiona, Victoria

I have been practising Qigong for thirty years on average about ten times per week. It was recommended as the best exercise program for my recovery from Post Viral Chronic Fatique Syndrome. After about six months of practice I decided I would do this for the rest of my life. Some of the other Chinese healing arts that I have used include acupuncture, massage and Chinese herbs. I am fitter and healthier now than I was thirty years ago.

I saw a demonstration by a Chinese Master of the Da Yan Wild Goose Qigong twenty-five years ago and thought it was the most amazing thing I had ever seen. Since then I have worked with books, DVDs and learned a short version, but it wasn't until I learned from Simon that I fully appreciated the depth, beauty and intricacies of the Da Yan.

It helps to balance the energy which flows through the meridians in our bodies and connects with the energy of the universe. It makes me feel fantastic and at peace. I often go to another place. I get to the end of a set and can't recall how I got there, even though I have done it perfectly. It keeps me flexible and fit, both in body and mind. Qigong had helped me to be mindful in everything I do. I have learned to be patient and understand things will work out for the best in due course.

In my opinion it is the best exercise anyone can do. As well as benefiting all the systems of the body (cardiovascular, muscular, skeletal, nervous, digestive, etc) it helps with energy (Qi) flow and is great for the mind. Use it or lose it!

Helen, New South Wales

I have been practising for three years and on an average I practise five times per week for about half an hour each session.

I was attending a workshop with Simon where we did some Qigong and then a meditation followed. I still remember Simon saying, "Return to the nothingness, because in the nothingness there is no disease, there is only nothing." I felt that space of nothingness and decided I would like to learn more Qigong to return to the nothingness.

I also currently practise Shiatsu which I consider a Chinese healing art and another form of Qigong known as Zhineng Qigong. Many years ago I learned Tai Chi which I did for several years.

Qigong is an exercise or movement that encourages the Qi (energy) to flow. I believe over a period of time it can help to clear stagnation in the meridian channels and improve the flow of Qi to all the internal organs, bones, blood etc. It definitely relaxes me and quietens my mind and I feel good doing something positive for myself.

I believe over a period of three years that my Qigong practice has helped me to be more peaceful and grounded. It is like my friend, so no matter where I go I can do it and it offers me stability. I believe it has helped with my circulation as I don't feel the cold as much in winter. It has also helped me with flexibility. Repeating the same routine each day is a good gauge as to how my body is feeling on that day. Just tuning into Qi and feeling the Qi helps with my Shiatsu practice.

Cathy, Victoria

I've been practising Qigong for about fifteen years. I practise five or six times a week.

I love the idea of training the mind, breath and body and finding balance and calm in my life. I also find the flowing movements suit my nature (I studied ballet for many years when young), because it is expressive of the beauty of the mind and body working in harmony. Qigong rewards persistence. I enjoy practising by myself, as well as teaching small groups. I maintain flexibility, can correct my posture and manage back and neck problems if I practise regularly.

The opportunity to learn from Master Chen in China was too good to miss. Before that visit, I hadn't heard of Da Yan Wild Goose Qigong. It was life-changing. Master Chen's revelation of his family's ancient practice was both humbling and exciting. It is such a beautiful form, both to watch and practise. I found the depth of twenty-seven generations of observing nature, refinement of the gestures and beauty of the movements to be profoundly moving. It was also physically and intellectually challenging to learn the form. I felt very fit by the end of the course!

I understand Qigong to be a practice whereby Qi is fostered and trained so that a state of harmony of mind, body and spirit is achieved. Qigong training promotes health, well-being and long life. You become aware through practising the inter-connectedness of the body and mind.

I feel strong, calm and balanced after practice. It takes me quietly through busy days, helps me to sleep and according to my husband, I 'glow' with energy post-practice.

I've benefitted in many ways from Qigong. In physical terms, I'm stronger, have better balance and coordination and my muscles and joints are moving freely. I can recognise symptoms of anxiety and use my practice to slow things down in my mind and body when it all gets too hectic. Qigong is also a wonderful aid to recovery from illness and surgery.

I've learned that you never stop learning! Qigong practice always has something new to teach you, to reveal to you if you are open to hearing and acting on the messages the mind and body are sending you. It's interesting that a practice that is focused on the self makes you more compassionate toward others. In nurturing the self, we give ourselves room to be more open-hearted and aware of other people. I enjoy meditation as part of Qigong. Partly because it balances 'action' with 'inaction' and because it focuses on the wholeness of human experience. I think too, that it is a practice for life, as it becomes an integral part of your day. I expect to be practising Qigong for the rest of my life.

Joy, Victoria

I have about eight years' experience in Qigong and in the last five years I have become very regular in my practice. I practise now at least three times a day on my own (Wild Goose just after 5am) and teach Qigong and Tai Chi five days per week. Fortunately I get at least one and a half hours' practice each day.

Learning Tai Chi in a musty hall in Sydney in 1988 gave me the first taste. My main incentive was for relaxation and health and in 2006 I became a fitness instructor and used Tai Chi in my classes. I studied a couple of courses and developed both my Qigong and Tai Chi from there. I practice and teach for my and others' relaxation and healing. I love how holistic and spiritual it is.
I believe Qigong it is an ancient art of working with energy to increase one's health, vitality and quality of life. It involves gentle exercise to stimulate and open the energy channels throughout the body, mind and spirit. It is accessible to all who are able and willing to engage in it. Qigong makes me feel fantastic- alive, centered and connected.

I am a doer, so taking action on a regular and ongoing basis with Wild Goose each morning gives me nurturing time and nourishment for myself! I am finding it easier to focus on present tasks, listen more and have a satisfying spiritual connection throughout the day. I'm frequently learning and being reminded that we are all one, that thoughts come and go and that the real thing is in the present experience. It helps me let go of 'wanting' and 'regretting'. I am engaging more with people I spend time with and tasks I enjoy. Life is somehow more flowing with the regular practice of Qigong, so most of all I am learning (work in progress) to let go of the notion that I am 'in control' and of being 'all responsible'.

The great mystery of Qigong is that the gentle 'doing' has a wonderful effect without needing to engage with the head. I trust that it is good for me. I relate to the journey of the geese, having moved so frequently in my life; the sense of leaving home on a journey and returning to home. The main part is the getting there and the leaving from there. While I am making a home where I am (in the last two years), it isn't just the physical location. It's the journey of life which is becoming more important, with the security of knowing my home is my base. The flock I move with is my mutual support.

Wendy, Tasmania

I have been practising Qigong for four years. When I'm in the groove, I practise it three times per week. Otherwise, I often go through the Wild Goose in my mind when I lie in bed.

Originally I was told about Qigong by a naturopath. I had fourth stage cancer and after attending my first retreat I knew that this was a great practice for me and that I would continue to explore it. Each time I do a retreat I feel more connected with the flow of energy in my body. It makes me feel vital and I seem to stand taller and am more alert. It really is wonderful.

Doing the movements in a Qigong sequence is about connecting with the subtle, internal flow of energy in the body. Initially it is difficult to perceive the connection points, but with time and practice these connections become stronger. It is one of the most beautiful forms of body/mind/energy connections I have experienced.

Qigong makes me feel centered and balanced. I find I am calmer and more able to be the mindful person I wish to be. I have learned that I can laugh and sing like a child, and feel liberated of the day-to-day challenges in life. I have learned that I can feel like a whole person.

Annie, New South Wales

I have been practising for eight years and I now practise on average six days a week.

I was in a lot of pain and had difficulty walking. My search on the internet and literature indicated Qigong could relieve this. I had used acupuncture on and off for about ten years whenever I twisted a knee or ankle and Chinese massage weekly for a couple of years for leg pain. The death of our dog left a huge void in my early mornings, when regardless of the weather, he insisted that we go out! Eventually I replaced our stroll around the beaches and headlands with the Wild Goose.

First, I see Qigong as a form of exercise. The Wild Goose in particular, with its 128 movements, includes a huge variety of movement and stances, together with essential breathing and mental applications. These all seem to encompass the requirements to maintain body strength, balance, and flexibility and mind power. As a philosophy it encompasses all the facets a person needs to live in harmony with nature, other people and oneself.

Qigong makes my blood flow, my body loosen, my joints become more flexible and my mind clearer and I feel ready to face the world. My balance and confidence have improved. I can now stand for the duration of the class without grasping for support.

Qigong practice is a continuous learning curve and Qigong's simplicity is what recommends it. You can practise without any equipment, anywhere, anytime, in any weather at no cost and you need no special clothing.

Margaret, New South Wales

I have been practising Qigong for five years now, and I average three practice sessions each week. I initially joined an exercise group run by U3A (University of the Third Age) where they worked from several different DVDs. Then Master Simon Blow visited and presented several workshops in the area and I was hooked. I have found it very helpful in maintaining flexibility and energy for more adventures. There is still so much to learn (I am now an octogenarian).

I studied with Grand Master Chen in China in 2009 and I found him a very interesting and delightful man whose family and students worked hard to pass on their knowledge. We worked hard, physically and mentally, to absorb so much in a short time. It was well worth the effort and a real privilege to have had the opportunity.

Qigong gives the body a chance to balance itself through a series of movements developed to promote the free flow of energy throughout the body and thus stimulate all systems. Qigong makes me feel calm and relaxed but remarkably energised. I might feel I'm too busy but if I start the day with my favourite, I find I get much more achieved. I've learned to keep an open mind and not to be afraid to explore new ideas.

I was wearing a brace on my right leg for osteo-arthritis in my knee but have abandoned that now. My knee still 'clicks' but now it has full movement and seldom do I have any discomfort.

I bless the day Simon Blow held some workshops in our country area and I went along. It was so worthwhile that when I found he was taking a group to China to learn Wild Goose I was lucky enough to be able to join in. What a wonderful time it was. I enjoyed the whole experience and loved the way passers-by would just join in practice sessions. The concept is obviously a complete way of life.

Shirley, New South Wales

CDs – by Simon Blow

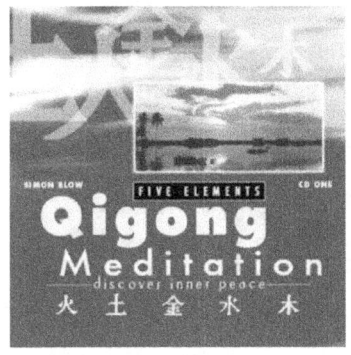

CD1: Five Elements Qigong Meditation

This CD is the perfect introduction to Qigong meditation (Neigong). **Track one** features a 30-minute heart-felt guided meditation to help bring love and light from the universe into your body. It harmonises the Five Elements – Fire, Earth, Metal, Water and Wood – with the corresponding organs of the body, respectively the heart, spleen, lungs, kidney and liver. This is one of the foundations of Chinese Qigong. Let Qigong Master Simon Blow help harmonise the elements of the universe with the energy of your body by using colour and positive images. **Track two** provides 30 minutes of relaxing music by inspiring composer Dale Nougher.

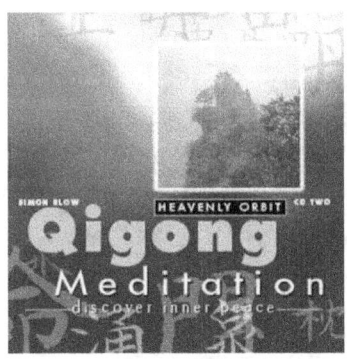

CD2: Heavenly Orbit Qigong Meditation

This CD is intended for the intermediate student. **Track one** takes you through a 30-minute guided meditation using your awareness to stimulate the energy centres around the body and open all the meridians. The circulation of Qi (Chi) around the Heavenly Orbit is one of the foundations of Chinese Qigong. The energy rising up the back 'Du' channel harmonises with the energy descending down the front 'Ren' channel, helping balance the energy of the body. Master Simon Blow guides you to open the energy centres of your own body to create harmony with the universe. **Track two** provides 30 minutes of relaxing music by Dale Nougher.

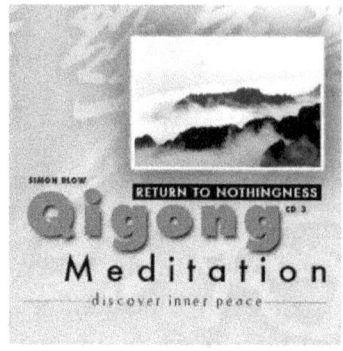

CD3: Return to Nothingness Qigong Meditation

This CD is intended for the advanced student and those wanting a healing night-practice. One of the aims of Qigong is to allow our internal energy (Qi) to harmonise with the external energy (Qi) allowing our consciousness to merge with the universe. When we enter into a deep sleep or meditation all the meridians start to open and much healing can take place. In this 20-minute guided meditation Simon Blow assists you in guiding your energy through your body and harmonising with the energy of the universe. Track two provides 30 minutes of healing music by Dale Nougher.

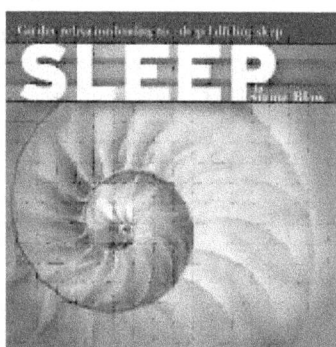

Sleep

Sleep is necessary to maintain life, alongside breathing, eating, drinking, and exercising of the mind and body. Without a good six to eight hours of sleep each night it can be hard to live a quality, balanced, fulfilling life. When we sleep it's a time to rest and rejuvenate the mind and body and to release the physical, mental and emotional stress that has built up during the day. This also helps uplift us spiritually.

It's a time to rest; it's time for a good night's sleep. Let Simon Blow's soothing voice, along with Dale Nougher's beautiful piano music and the natural sounds of the ocean, help guide you to release the tension of the day and enable you to enter a deep, fulfilling sleep.

Book/DVD sets – by Simon Blow

"About 18 months ago I started to practise Qigong as I knew that it would improve my health. I needed to do it regularly, ideally every day, but being in a rural area presented logistical problems. I discovered Simon's DVD and commenced daily practice. The great advantage for me was that I didn't have to travel to classes and could do them whenever I felt like it. Since that time I have noticed great improvement in my overall wellbeing. It has helped me to reinvent my clinical practice as a holistic massage practitioner. A number of my clients now have Simon's DVD and I feel this is helping them to both improve their health and well being, and to empower themselves." **Robin Godson-King (Holistic Massage Practitioner)**

(Each set contains a DVD plus a book that provides diagrams and instructions for the movements contained on the DVD. The book also includes interesting reading about the practice of Qigong as well as inspirational stories.)

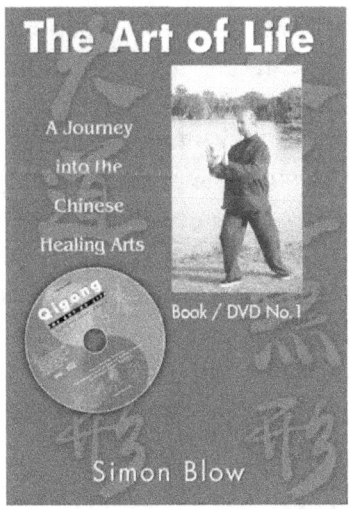

The Art of Life

'The Art of Life' presents the Qigong styles that were taught to me in Australia: the Taiji Qigong Shibashi, which I learned as an instructor with the Australian Academy of Tai Chi from 1990 to 1995; and the Ba Duan Jin standing form, commonly known as the Eight Pieces of Brocade, taught to me in 1996 by Sifu John Dolic in Sydney.

This is the perfect introduction to this ancient art and is suitable for new and continuing students of all ages. The book follows the DVD and contains three sections: **1. Warm up** – gentle movements loosen all the major joints of the body, lubricating the tendons and helping increase blood and energy circulation. It is beneficial for most arthritic conditions; **2. Ba Duan Jin or Eight Pieces of Brocade** – this is the best known and most widely practised form of Qigong throughout the world, also known as Daoist Yoga. The movements stretch all the major muscles, massage organs and open the meridians of the body; **3. Taiji Qigong Shibashi** – this popular practice is made up of eighteen flowing movements. The gentle movements harmonise the mind, body and breath. Total running time: 55 minutes.

"Tai Chi Qigong is a gentle way of exercising the whole body and provides long-term benefits. I recommend it to my patients as an effective way of improving muscle tone and joint mobility. Those who practise regularly have fewer problems with their muscles and joints and often report an increased sense of health and wellbeing. This is an excellent video with clear and simple instruction."

Roman Maslak. B.A. (Hons), D.O. Osteopath

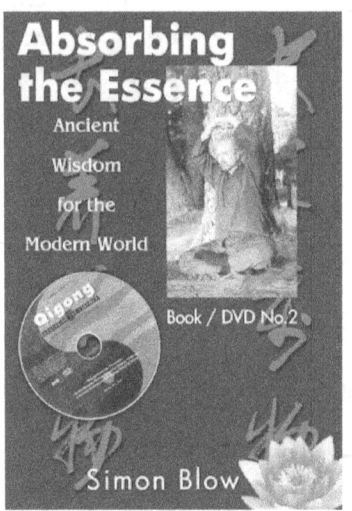

Absorbing the Essence

'Absorbing the Essence' comprises the Qigong cultivation techniques that were taught to me by Grand Master Zhong Yunlong in 1999 and 2000 at Wudangshan or Wudang Mountain. Wudang is one of the sacred Daoist Mountains of China and is renowned for the development of Taiji.

This DVD and book is for the intermediate student and for people with experience in meditation. It contains three sections: **1. Warm up** – the same as in The Art of Life DVD; **2. Wudang Longevity Qigong** – this sequence of gentle, flowing movements stimulates the Heavenly Orbit, absorbing the primordial energy from the environment and letting the negativity dissolve into the distance; **3. Sitting Ba Duan Jin** – this 30-minute sequence includes eight sections with exercises to stimulate different organs and meridians of the body. It is practised in a seated position on a chair or cushion – ideal for people who have discomfort whilst standing. These practices originated from the famous Purple Cloud Monastery at the sacred Wudang Mountain in China. Total running time: 60 minutes.

"Simon Blow of Australia has twice travelled (1999, 2000) to Mt Wudang Shan Daoist Wushu College to learn Taiji Hunyuan Zhuang (Longevity) Qigong and Badajin Nurturing Life Qigong and through his study has absorbed the essence of these teachings. Therefore, I specially grant Simon the authority to teach these, spreading the knowledge of these Qigong methods he has learnt at Mt Wudang to contribute to the wellbeing of the human race. May the Meritorious Deeds Be Infinite."

Grand Master Zhong Yunlong, Daoist Priest and Director,
Mt Wudang Shan Taoist Wushu College, China, September 24, 2000.

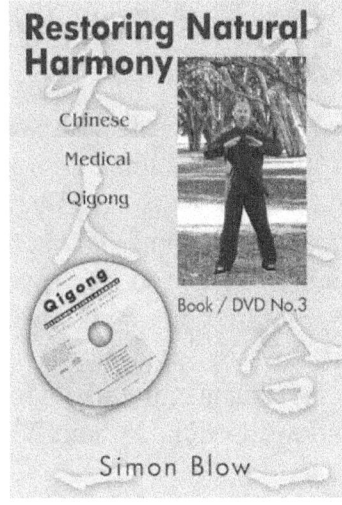

Restoring Natural Harmony
Chinese Medical Qigong
Qigong
Book / DVD No.3
Simon Blow

Restoring Natural Harmony

This DVD and book is for the advanced student or for the person wanting to learn specific Traditional Chinese Medicine self-healing exercises. Each section works on a different organ meridian system of the body – Spleen, Lungs, Kidney, Liver and Heart – which relate to the Five Elements – Earth, Metal, Water, Wood and Fire. Guigen Qigong originated from Dr Xu Hongtao, a Qigong Specialist Doctor from the Xiyuan Hospital in Beijing. These internal exercises help regulate the meridian system bringing harmony to mind, body and spirit. Total running time: 75 minutes.

"Simon Blow first visited our hospital in 2002. I was impressed with his knowledge and commitment to Qigong. He returned in 2004 to study Chinese Medical Qigong. Simon is a gifted teacher: he has the rare ability to inspire others and impart to them the healing benefits of Qigong."
Dr Xu Hongtao, Qigong and Tuina Department, Xiyuan Hospital Beijing, China.

"This DVD – the third by the impressively qualified Sydney-based Simon Blow – serves two purposes. Firstly, it is so attractively produced that the curious would surely be induced to investigate further. Secondly, for those already practising, it provides a mnemonic device much more useful than a series of still pictures." **Review by Adyar Bookshop, Sydney 2005.**

These are not medical devices and should not be used to replace any existing medical treatment. Always consult with your health provider if uncertain.

Da Yan Wild Goose Qigong
The first 64 movements

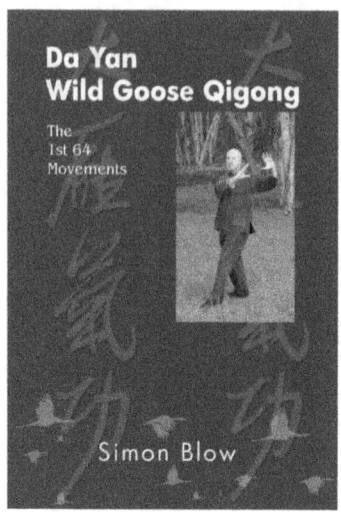

'Da Yan' translates to 'great bird' and is an ancient cultivation practice originating from the Jin Dynasty about 1700 years ago. Daoist Masters from the sacred Kunlun Mountains, in the Northern Himalayan area in south-west China, would observe the migrating geese which descended in this area each year. They would mimic the movements of these great birds and started to developed the Da Yan Wild Goose Qigong system.

Its healing and spiritual legacy was passed down through many generations; however Dayan Qigong was withheld from the general public until 1978. Then 27th lineage holder Grand Master Yang Mei Jung (1895-2002) decided to teach this ancient Qigong practice and share its healing benefits to improve the quality of life of all people.

The 1st 64 movement set deals primary with the 'post-natal body' relating to the energy that one gathers after birth. The movements representing the flight of wild geese are slow, graceful movements and strong, quick movements designed to release stale Qi and to gather fresh Qi, helping to restore balance and stimulate the entire energy system of the body.

'I've benefitted in many ways from Qigong. In physical terms, I'm stronger, have better balance and coordination and my muscles and joints are moving freely. I can recognise symptoms of anxiety and use my practice to slow things down in my mind and body when it all gets too hectic. Qigong is also a wonderful aid to recovery from illness and surgery.' **Joy**

'I am finding it easier to focus on present tasks, listen more and have a satisfying spiritual connection throughout the day.' **Wendy**

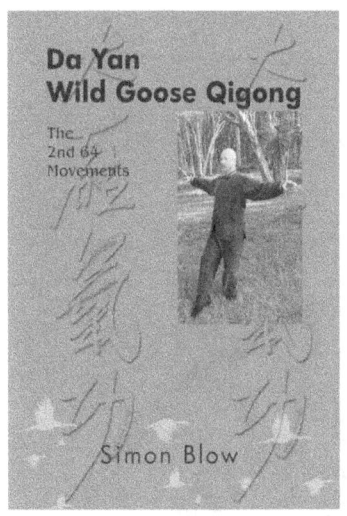

Da Yan Wild Goose Qigong
The second 64 movements

From ancient times, Qigong was an important component of the Chinese medical health system, and developed to help improve people's quality of life. The art of Qigong consists primarily of meditation, relaxation, physical movement, mind-body integration and breathing exercises. When the mind and body come into a state of balance, stress is reduced and there is an increase in health and longevity.

The 2nd 64 movement set of Da Yan Wild Goose Qigong deals primarily with the 'pre-natal body', which refers to the energy we gather from the universe and from our ancestors before birth. Having dredged the channels in the 1st 64 movement set, the 2nd 64 movement set is designed to clear the channels to absorb fresh Qi, expel stale Qi and to restore organ balance. The twisting, stretching, bending and pressing movements produce stronger Qi fields and intensify the circulation through the energy channels. In the 2nd 64 movement set, the Goose embarks on a great journey and flies out from this world to the edge of the Milky Way to pick herbs or gather pre-natal Qi from the core of the universe. It then flies back to this world to share this healing energy with humanity.

'Simon's greatest gift is his ability to make complex concepts so accessible to all people. His teaching is so clear yet so simple and profound that everybody feels included and encouraged to advance further. As a Qigong teacher this is what I hope to achieve in the future.' **Sylvia**

'Qigong has taught me to be more aware of how and what I feel; to listen to my body and to be kinder to myself. My Qigong practice has also given me the confidence to teach with diligence, and to inspire my students. Each day is a wonderful experience; life is good.' **Cherel**

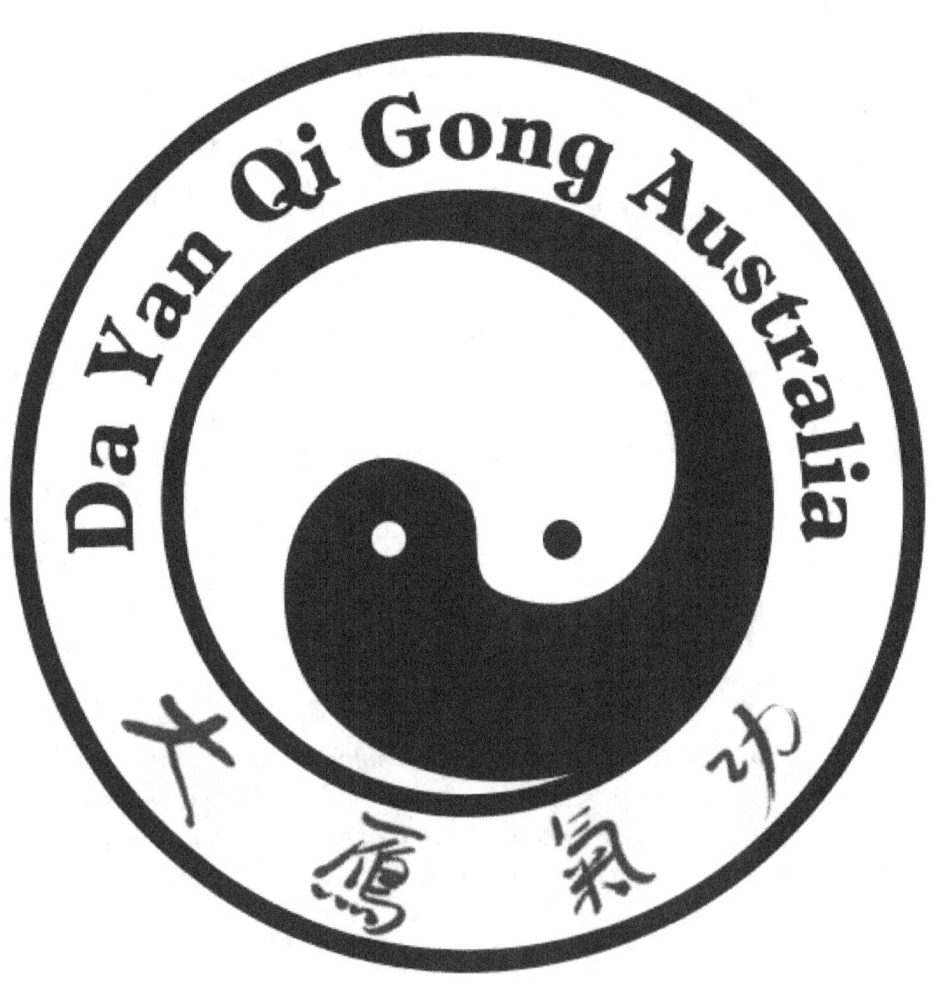

☯ Simon Blow Qigong 信思

— for better health and inner peace —

To order products or for more information on:
- Regular classes in Sydney for new and continuing students
- Workshops or if you would be interested in helping organise a workshop in your local area
- Residential Qigong and Meditation retreats
- China Qigong Study Tours for students and advanced training
- Talks, corporate classes, training and presentations
- Wholesale enquiries

Please contact:

Simon Blow
PO Box 446
Summer Hill, NSW 2130
Sydney Australia

Ph: +61 (0)2 9559 8153

Web: **www.simonblowqigong.com**

CDs and Book/DVDs can be ordered online and shipped nationally and internationally.

Bibliography

Yang Meijun, *Wild Goose Qigong*. China: China Science and Technology Press. 1991

Liu TJ, Chen KW et al. (eds) *Chinese Medical Qigong*. London: Singing Dragon. 2010.

Ni Hua-Ching. *Esoteric Tao Teh Ching*. California: Seven Star Communications Group, Inc., 1992.

Ni Hua-Ching. *The Gentle Path of Spiritual Progress*. California: Shrine of the Eternal Breath of Tao, 1987

Ellis, Wiseman, Boss. *Grasping the Wind*. Massachusetts: Paradigm Publications , 1989

Yang, Jwing-Ming. *The Root of Chinese Qigong*, Massachusetts: YMAA Publication Centre, 1997.
Blow Simon. *The Art of Life*. Sydney: Genuine Wisdom Centre, 2010
Blow Simon. *Absorbing the Essence*. Sydney: Genuine Wisdom Centre, 2010
Blow Simon. *Restoring Natural Harmony*. Sydney: Genuine Wisdom Centre, 2010
Basic Theory of Traditional Chinese Medicine. China: Publishing House of Shanghai University of Traditional Chinese Medicine, 2002.

Liu, Qingshan. *Chinese Fitness*. Massachusetts: YMAA Publication Centre, 1997.

Magpie Goose People story Copyright © George Milpurrurru

Websites

www.wikipedia.org
www.esotericastrologer.org
www.eng.taoism.org.hk
www.dierinbeeld.nl/animal_files/birds/goose/
www.egreenway.com/taichichuan/goose.htm

Meridian charts originally sourced from Basic Theory of Traditional Chinese Medicine. China: Publishing House of Shanghai University of Traditional Chinese Medicine. 1988

Meridian Acupoints originally sourced
www.cgicm.ca/cn
www.en.tcm-china
www.acupuncture.com
www.thedaoofdragonball.com
www.compassionatedragon.com
www.ttpacupuncture.com
www.shen-nong.com
www.buzzle.com